Praise for
The Sustainable Mediterranean Diet Cookbook

"If there were a trifecta for cookbooks, *The Sustainable Mediterranean Diet Cookbook* would be a winning bet for the planet and your kitchen. Deanna and Serena bring you well-crafted, healthy recipes, seasonal swaps, and tips to make your kitchen sustainable. Plus, their healthy kitchen hacks will have you cooking instinctually like a pro!"

— Lari Robling, author of the internationally acclaimed *Endangered Recipes*, independent radio producer and writer, and James Beard nominee for Best Food Radio

"*The Sustainable Mediterranean Diet Cookbook* is not only delicious, but a nutritious collection of recipes that are good for your health and the environment, and easy on your pocketbook. The Mediterranean diet has long been known as one of the healthiest diets in the world because the people who enjoy this delicious cuisine are super healthy and free of many chronic diseases. If there is one diet plan that is universally good for health and the planet, it's the sustainable Mediterranean diet. Everyone needs this cookbook by these very talented registered dietitian nutritionists who know the importance of delicious food, sustainability, protecting the planet, and eating a plant-forward diet for good health."

— Kathleen Zelman, MPH, RDN, owner of No Nonsense Nutrition and host of True Health Initiative's *True Health Revealed* podcast

"So much more than a cookbook, [*The Sustainable Mediterranean Diet Cookbook*] is a path to sustainability and health through delicious, nutritious food. The top 10 eco-friendly kitchen guidelines are approachable and innovative. Serena and Deanna provide crave-worthy Mediterranean-style recipes that are simple and tasty."

—Chef Abbie Gellman, MS, RDN, CDN, author of *The Mediterranean DASH Diet Cookbook* and *Instant Pot Mediterranean Diet Cookbook*

"In *The Sustainable Mediterranean Diet Cookbook*, Serena Ball and Deanna Segrave-Daly share resourceful and sustainable cooking tips inspired by Mediterranean cuisine. These creative, easy recipes put flavor first and are built around ingredients that nourish both people and the planet."

—Kelly LeBlanc, MLA, RD, LDN, director of nutrition at Oldways

THE Sustainable Mediterranean Diet COOKBOOK

Also by Serena Ball, MS, RD, and Deanna Segrave-Daly, RD

The 30-Minute Mediterranean Diet Cookbook
Easy Everyday Mediterranean Diet Cookbook

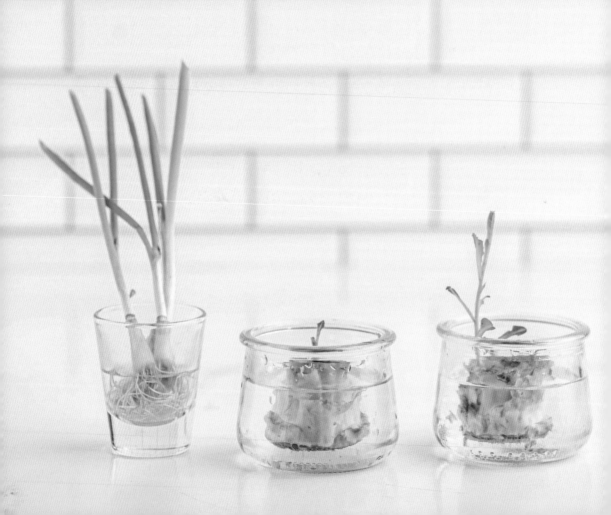

THE Sustainable Mediterranean Diet
COOKBOOK

*More Than 100 Easy, Healthy Recipes
to Reduce Food Waste,
Eat in Season, and Help the Earth*

**Serena Ball, MS, RD,
and Deanna Segrave-Daly, RD**

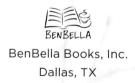

BenBella Books, Inc.
Dallas, TX

Many of the designations used by manufacturers and sellers to distinguish their products are claimed as trademarks. Where those designations appear in this book and BenBella Books was aware of a trademark claim, the designations have been printed in initial capital letters.

The Sustainable Mediterranean Diet Cookbook copyright © 2022 by Deanna Segrave-Daly and Serena Ball

Photographs by Elise Cellucci

BenBella Books, Inc.
10440 N. Central Expressway
Suite 800
Dallas, TX 75231
benbellabooks.com
Send feedback to feedback@benbellabooks.com

BenBella is a federally registered trademark.

Printed in the United States of America
10 9 8 7 6 5 4 3 2 1

Library of Congress Control Number: 2022013471
ISBN 9781637741542 (paperback)
ISBN 9781637741559 (electronic)

Editing by Claire Schulz
Copyediting by Karen Wise
Proofreading by Amy Zarkos and Isabelle Rubio
Indexing by Debra Bowman
Text design and composition by Kit Sweeney
Cover design by Sarah Avinger
Cover photography by Elise Cellucci
Printed by Versa Press

**Special discounts for bulk sales are available.
Please contact bulkorders@benbellabooks.com.**

Contents

Introduction

Welcome to our Mediterranean table. It's overflowing with simple but delicious dishes rich in colorful vegetables, lentils and beans, olives and olive oil, succulent fruits, herbs and spices, whole grains, crunchy seeds and nuts, briny fish and shellfish, yogurt and cheeses, eggs, and occasionally chicken and meat. While the origins of the "Mediterranean diet" began in the 1960s after nutrition researchers found that working-class communities in Greece and Italy had low incidence of heart disease, the term has evolved to encompass the similar eating patterns found in the lands surrounding the Mediterranean Sea. These countries include Italy, Greece, Turkey, Syria, Lebanon, Israel, Egypt, Libya, Tunisia, Algeria, Morocco, Spain, and southern France. People from these cultures often eat with purpose; they slow down and enjoy meals with good cheer and sociability when they sit at a table. With decades of solid nutrition research to support it, this lifestyle continues to appeal to people of all ages who like to eat (we bet you're one of those).

As you sit down at this table, you may notice something else: everything here is not only good for *you*, but also good for the *planet*.

That's right: while we love the Mediterranean diet for its health benefits and fabulous flavors, it also provides an easy template for eco-friendly food shopping, preparation, and cooking. In fact, experts have deemed it one of the *best* eating plans for protecting the planet's resources. So if you're looking for "climate cuisine," look no further.

But if you've ever found yourself standing in the grocery store wondering where to start with the Mediterranean diet, or even wondering if it's worth it to worry about one more thing (after all, you're *already* considering price, nutrition, and most importantly, taste), we can help! This book is designed to make the Mediterranean lifestyle easy and fun. Taking a few small steps at a time can make an impact—in lowering your grocery bill, reducing your electricity use, and improving your health *and* the Earth.

If your doctor told you to follow the Mediterranean diet and you grabbed this cookbook, the recipes here will help you sit down to savor sustainable meals you'll enjoy making for yourself and your family. You may even want to start cooking for your friends—a leisurely, sociable dinner is the Mediterranean way!

This is our third Mediterranean diet cookbook. We are registered dietitians and busy moms, Serena from the Midwest with five kids and Deanna from Philly with a teenager. These are recipes we actually feed our families and friends—and we have for over a decade. They are not necessarily traditional recipes, and we are not experts in Mediterranean cultural cuisines, compared to those who are natives of those regions. But the dishes you will find here are rich in ingredients originating from the Mediterranean. Over the years, we have traveled to several Mediterranean countries and fallen in love with the flavors there. Our hope is that you, too, will embrace the spice za'atar, use olive oil as your main fat source, and try cooking with little fishes and other Mediterranean-style foods—many of which are made or grown by Mediterranean-descended families in our neck of the woods, and most likely yours too!

In "Eating Eco-Friendly the Mediterranean Diet Way," you'll find our *Top 10 Eco-Friendly Kitchen Guidelines* for shopping, prepping, cooking, eating, and storing food. Every recipe follows at least one of these guidelines. And because eliminating food waste is a huge part of a more sustainable diet, we also share a *Use It or Lose It* section with helpful suggestions on what to do with leftover ingredients (like that handful of fresh herbs or half can of tomato sauce).

Then, you'll find more than 100 sustainable, family-friendly, time- and money-saving recipes—developed by dietitians—featuring Mediterranean ingredients that can easily be found in regular grocery stores. These appealing and uncomplicated recipes are flexible, as many provide options to modify according to your needs. Every single recipe features *Healthy Kitchen Hack*s with shortcuts, ingredient substitutions, energy-saving ideas, and helpful cooking tips. Most recipes have been double- and triple-tested by real home cooks across the country from our TeaspoonofSpice.com blog community. Their comments, reviews, and tips appear throughout the book.

If you eat gluten-free, dairy-free, egg-free, nut-free, vegetarian, or vegan, check the recipe notes—there's something here just for you! The Mediterranean diet is a plant-forward way of eating that lends itself naturally to vegetarian diets (and trimming meat consumption is an aspect of climate cuisine). That said, we know there are many meat-lovers out there who are also trying to eat more plant-based meals while being eco-conscious. Our seafood, meat, and poultry recipes showcase more sustainable protein choices so you can still enjoy the foods you love while making changes for the better.

Finally, we share four complete five-day meal plans: Gluten-Free, Vegetarian, Seafood Twice a Week, and Meatless Monday.

We hope this book brings a bit of Mediterranean sunshine to your own kitchen—wherever you're located—while also helping you make a positive impact on the Earth. Thank you for inviting us in!

Serena and Deanna

Eating Eco-Friendly the Mediterranean Way

The dishes, spices, local ingredients, and combinations of foods eaten daily by people in Mediterranean regions can vary greatly, but the similarities of eating patterns are what have come to define the Mediterranean diet. These commonalities include olive oil as the main fat, greater amounts of whole grains, beans and legumes, nuts and seeds, fruits, vegetables, fish a few times a week, fermented dairy foods like yogurt and cheese frequently, eggs often along with some poultry, and infrequent meat and sweets. Water and wine (for those who drink alcohol) are the main beverages.

Why Go Med?

Researchers have discovered many health benefits associated with the Mediterranean diet. (We prefer the word "lifestyle" because "diet" can bring to mind deprivation or restriction—but here, the term should be understood simply as a way of eating.) Studies show people who follow the Mediterranean diet generally have less risk of developing Alzheimer's disease, dementia, and other psychiatric disorders, and in a 2010 study by researchers at the Bordeaux Population Health Research Center, "Mediterranean Diet and Cognitive Function in Older Adults," the authors concluded that close adherence to the Mediterranean diet may help prevent cognitive decline. Additionally, the Mediterranean diet has long been associated with lower risk of cardiovascular diseases and more recently with lower rates of arthritis, asthma, cancer, cardiovascular disease, diabetes, high blood pressure, and high cholesterol. Studies also show that people who follow a Mediterranean lifestyle overall have lower blood pressure, lower blood lipids, and a lower weight. As a result, health professionals for decades have encouraged people to adopt a Mediterranean lifestyle to protect their health.

More recently, a 2019 report by leading health and sustainability experts, published in the distinguished medical journal *The Lancet*, showed that the Mediterranean diet is one of the best ways to eat for the health of the Earth. And when you think of the foods of the Mediterranean diet, maybe that's no surprise! Typical Mediterranean diet dishes feature lots of beans and legumes, which have a small carbon footprint and also nourish the soil—and that healthy soil can then be used to grow more crops. Eating fruits and vegetables when they're in season is the norm. The sea and its local bounty, including smaller fishes that are found in greater supply, is a prime source of protein. Locally produced dairy products, especially cheese and yogurt, are key ingredients. Finally, the diet involves smaller amounts of land animal–protein foods, and using the entire animal, including the offal, is also typical. But overall, this eating pattern is primarily based on plants—be they fresh and local, frozen, or canned.

If you need any more convincing, for many years running, after reviewing 40 different diet plans, a panel of health experts and *U.S. News & World Report* have ranked the Mediterranean diet as the best diet overall, both for its benefits and for how easy it is to follow. Additionally, it's one of only three eating patterns recommended in the current edition of the government nutrition experts' U.S. Dietary Guidelines for Americans.

Top 10 Eco-Friendly Kitchen Guidelines

So, how can you follow the Mediterranean lifestyle *and* have a more eco-friendly kitchen? Luckily, as we mentioned earlier, they are basically the same! To help you take your climate cuisine to the next level, we've outlined ten realistic guidelines to keep in mind any time you shop for, prepare, cook, and store food. Each recipe in this book showcases one, if not several, of these sustainability tips. So, just by making a handful of the recipes in this book, you're helping make a difference, deliciously!

This is by no means an exhaustive list, nor are we expecting you to adopt them all. But adapting at least one guideline into a habit—in your own Mediterranean lifestyle— can help you be sustainable wherever *you* live.

1. Reduce food waste

When we toss any food in the trash, we don't just create food waste, we also waste all the energy and water it took to grow, harvest, transport, and package that food. And once it gets to a landfill, it rots and creates methane, a greenhouse gas. Just about every recipe in this book highlights specific ways to cut back on food waste. Here are the highlights and principles we follow again and again:

Use up the entire herb. Both the leaves *and* the stems of parsley, cilantro, and usually mint and basil can be finely chopped and thrown into recipes and salads; the tender stems add crunch and texture. Cilantro stems are actually sweeter than the leaves.

Stalks and stems are tasty. Broccoli and cauliflower stalks and cabbage cores can be chopped up and used just as you use the rest of the veggie. They are often the best-tasting part; for instance, broccoli stalks are sweeter and more tender than the florets.

Keep skins on. Most of the powerful antioxidants found in plants are located right beneath the skins (so plants can more efficiently repair themselves if attacked by insects). When you remove the peel on an apple, carrot, or beet, you lose some of the nutritional benefits. So keep the peels on your potatoes, and (since one of our testers asked!) don't peel your zucchini either. As long as the peels aren't super tough (like acorn squash), you can safely eat them.

Save the scraps. Almost all parts of veggies, including those we don't eat—from onion skins to carrot ends to corn cobs—can be saved in a freezer container for making Veggie Scraps Broth (page 120).

Savor the seeds. Roast the seeds from pumpkins and other winter squashes like butternut and acorn squash. For an easy recipe, check out our Toasted Squash Seeds and Cheese Board (page 61).

Enjoy the whole citrus. Before cutting and juicing limes and lemons for a recipe, zest the peel—if you don't use it in the recipe, it can be frozen to use later on. Store any extra juice in a refrigerator jar or pour into ice cube trays and freeze. Toss the zested peel and juiced flesh down the garbage disposal to freshen your kitchen, or compost them.

Compost. Learn how to set up a simple compost pile in your yard, then start a garden or donate the compost to a neighbor or community garden. Or, find a local composting program that picks up curbside.

Buy "ugly" produce. Search out fruit and veggies that look less than perfect—they taste just as good, and if you don't buy them, they will likely get tossed. Ask your grocer to start a "reduced-price fruit bin," especially for overripe bananas, slightly bruised apples, and other "misfit" fruit.

Store produce properly. Keep your fruits and veggies in the right spots in the refrigerator—or on the counter. See the How to Store Produce box on page 7.

Enjoy more frozen fruits and vegetables. Because frozen foods last a long time, there's less chance they'll wind up like some fresh foods—forgotten until they go bad in the fridge and have to be tossed. And since produce is frozen at the peak of ripeness, freezing locks in nutrients that can get lost in the long transport journeys of fresh produce.

Treat spice nice. Buy only what you need to use up within a year; mark the purchase date on each. Spices don't spoil, but they do lose their flavor over time. If older than a year, use at least ¼ teaspoon more than the called-for amount until that spice is gone. Whole spices last much longer; so try grinding your own from whole. Avoid storing spices near the stove as heat zaps taste and aroma.

How to Store Produce

Store at room temperature on the countertop *Refrigerate once ripe **Refrigerate to extend storage if needed	Avocados,* bananas, basil (in water like a bouquet), citrus fruits (grapefruit, lemons, limes, oranges),** eggplant,* mangoes,* pears,* pineapples,* stone fruits (apricots, nectarines, peaches, plums)*, tomatoes*
Store in the refrigerator	Apples, avocadoes (ripe), beets, bell peppers, berries, broccoli, cabbage, carrots, cauliflower, celery, cherries, corn, cucumbers, fresh herbs (except basil; wash first, trim, place stems in jar with 1 inch water, tightly cover), fresh beans (green beans, snap peas, snow peas), scallions (green onions), leafy greens, melons, mushrooms, radishes, summer squash
Store in the pantry or a cool, dark place *Refrigerate in hot weather	Garlic, ginger root, onions, potatoes (avoid storing near onions to prevent potatoes from sprouting sooner), sweet potatoes,* winter squash

2. Eat in season

There's certainly something to be said for keeping farmers around the world in business growing fruit all year. But unless you live in a warm climate, buying strawberries in winter usually means that fruit has traveled a lot of miles before the produce gets to your plate. Buying in-season produce often means that food was grown nearby and thus cuts down on the greenhouse gas emissions associated with transporting food. Produce that travels further can also lose vitamin content along the way. Try eating according to the following seasons *most* of the time; or try doing so for a week at a time a few times each season. This exercise may make you want to stock up and freeze a few more summer berries to have on hand when winter comes. (Of course, frozen fruits/veggies are in season all year!) Here's a seasonal guide:

- **Winter:** Potatoes, carrots, beets, cabbage, greenhouse-grown lettuce, citrus fruit, apples, pears, onions, leeks, dates, kiwifruit, pomegranate, parsnips, sweet potatoes

- **Spring:** Asparagus, peas, berries, artichokes, many lettuces (like butter, Bibb, Boston, mâche, and mesclun), spinach, dandelion greens, rhubarb, fiddlehead ferns, snow peas, watercress, morel mushrooms, radishes, scallions

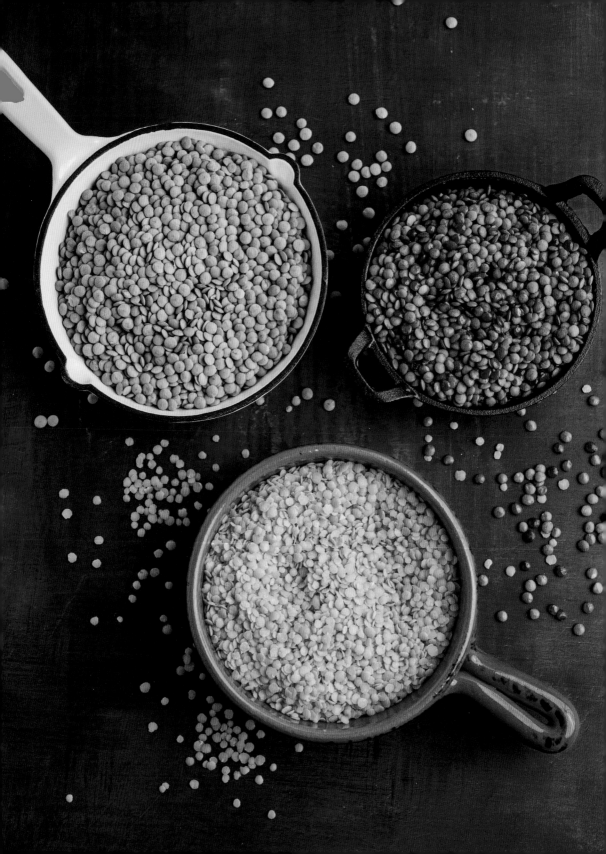

- **Summer:** Peaches, plums, berries, tomatoes, green beans, peas, figs, bell peppers, hot peppers, cucumbers, melons (like watermelon and cantaloupe), eggplant, jackfruit, passionfruit, zucchini, summer squash, tomatillo
- **Fall:** Broccoli, Brussels sprouts, kohlrabi, winter squashes, apples, pears, grapes, garlic, onions, Jerusalem artichokes, pomegranate, quince, persimmons, turnips, romaine lettuce, Swiss chard, kale

3. Buy more sustainable staple crops

Many pantry staple foods are adaptable to different growing climates and can even help the soil where they're grown. Some of them can be grown year-round and are very shelf-stable, meaning they're always in season for you!

Eat more legumes. Lentils, dried peas, chickpeas, and beans actually regenerate the soil. And without healthy soil, we can't have tasty plants or healthy animals, for that matter. Take advantage of the variety (and low price!) of both dried beans and canned beans. See our Everyday Pot of Lentils on page 170 for recipe inspiration.

Mix in mushrooms. The humble mushroom can be grown year-round almost anywhere (even indoors), requiring only a tiny amount of water and land. Add finely chopped mushrooms to ground meat to extend and make more burgers, meatloaf, or meatballs (see Spiced Ground Beef over Lemon Hummus, page 231). Or, make them the star of your plate in vegetarian meals like our Roasted Thyme Mushrooms over Parmesan Polenta Squares on page 193.

Snack on seeds. You'll notice that we use more seeds than nuts in this book (for example, in our Vanilla and Fruit Seeded Granola Bars on page 66). Seeds (and peanuts, which are not nuts but legume seeds) typically use significantly less water to grow compared to many tree nuts, are drought-resistant, and provide food for bees and birds. Sesame seeds are a big staple in Middle Eastern cuisines; they star in the spice blend za'atar (try it in our Cheesy Broccoli Greens Soup with Za'atar, page 121). Store seeds in your freezer for maximum freshness and to last longer.

Eat oats often. Oats are generally considered a low-input crop, meaning they require fewer resources to grow compared to other crops. They are also frequently used in crop rotations with lentils, which can help improve soil health. Try the Fig-Orange Overnight Oats on page 31.

4. Look before you cook

Before you go to the store because there's "no food in the house," explore your pantry. If you've stocked pasta, canned tomatoes, canned vegetables, olive oil, and a few spices, you're covered for dinner. And for dessert, check the freezer: you may have the makings for frozen fruit shakes or smoothies!

Make a pantry meal. Here's what we stock in our kitchens to make sure we always have the makings of a full meal on hand:

- Dried pasta, beans, bulgur, couscous, barley, farro, oats
- Canned tomatoes, beans, vegetables, fruits, olives, capers
- Canned seafood and chicken
- Frozen fruits and vegetables (lots of them!)
- Frozen fish
- Refrigerated condiments, yogurt, cheese, eggs

Check the fridge. Dibs and dabs in the refrigerator can be used up—check out our Use It or Lose It List on page 21. And leftovers can be repurposed and stretched by serving them on top of toast, a baked potato, quick-cooking barley, or even a bed of herbs or greens. Try our Spicy Red Lentil and Chorizo Stew on page 238.

Creatively substitute . . . everything! Sometimes a recipe becomes even better when you substitute an ingredient because you don't have what's listed. Our recipes often have several suggestions for an ingredient. No need to go buy fresh basil for a recipe if you already have cilantro, especially if the cilantro is starting to go limp. (When we call for fresh herbs, you can often substitute their dried counterparts as well!)

Add water. Speaking of limp cilantro—or scallions, carrots, celery, radishes, or other sad veggies—these and many others can be revived by soaking them in clean, cold water. First, wash the veggies, then snip off the stems or tips so the vegetables have a fresh way to absorb water; soak for 15 minutes to an hour, depending on how wilted. Use them right away, or drain and place in a container and back in the fridge to use within a day or two.

Make fruit sauce. For sad fruit, make our Ugly Fruit Jam (page 259) to pour over yogurt, ricotta cheese, or crusty bread. Or follow that same jam recipe, add an apple or two, and puree for any-fruit applesauce, or use a food dehydrator to make fruit leather. (You can find food dehydrators at online garage sales, like Serena did.)

5. Buy local

As with buying in-season, buying local (when possible) limits how far food has to travel before it reaches your plate. Plus you will be supporting the efforts of farmers and ranchers in your area, which in turn helps increase the health of the soil and the air near you. It's rare to find a farmer or rancher who doesn't protect the soil, since they know it's their biggest asset; well-supported farmers can stay in business longer preserving farm/range lands and preventing city sprawl with accompanying air pollution. (This is a generalization, but you get the idea!)

Ask for local products. Talk to the folks at the customer service counter of your local grocery store. Often local products are flagged on the shelves or even have their own aisle.

Support farmers' markets. They're a terrific way to buy local, and you'll cut down on packaging since most produce is sold loose at these markets. And striking up a conversation with farmers can lead to discussions about what is coming into season, so you can plan, and the farmers can sell more of what they grow.

Sign up for a CSA share. A community-supported agriculture (CSA) plan isn't only sustainable, it's an adventure! Many CSA offerings contain varieties of fruits, vegetables, and herbs you can't buy in a grocery store. Substitute them into many of our recipes—ask the farmer how!

Challenge yourself to buy products from within a 100-mile radius. Try it for a week and see what you discover. This includes items like, but not limited to, locally produced condiments, household products, breads, honey, meat, and dairy foods. Ask around at the farmers' market (especially the market organizer) to see what other farmers and their patrons are finding beyond what the market sells.

6. Grow (some of) your food

It is a satisfying and joyous occasion to sit down to eat even a small salad of lettuce and herbs you grew yourself. Homegrown veggies also don't require any gas or other transportation costs to travel to your plate; plus, not a bit of packaging is needed. That said, it can be intimidating to rip up a patch of your lawn and try to get something to grow. And that's assuming you have a lawn! You might be working with a balcony or patio, or even a sunny windowsill. The key is to start small, or even hydroponically.

Start with herbs. Purchase potted herbs from your grocery store or a local nursery. Once you get the hang of taking care of them, you can expand your collection by planting herb seeds in pots. (See our Healthy Kitchen Hack on page 76.) There's nothing like the taste of herbs snipped and added to a dish minutes before eating it. And bonus: any indoor plant helps clean the air in your home.

Recycle and grow. Deanna doesn't have the best luck growing houseplants, but she's found it a snap to regrow scallions from store-bought scallion roots and romaine lettuce from the bottoms. (See our Healthy Kitchen Hack on page 70.)

Garden in small spaces. Plant in large outdoor pots or on a small section of lawn. Get inspired by a gardening blogger or a neighbor who's got a green thumb, or call your local county extension agent. Every county has one, and they can be super helpful in teaching you about your local resources and even what types of vegetables will grow best in your soil.

Make a spot for your compost. If you compost, you're already making free dirt. Start a small garden to use that dirt or simply camouflage your compost bin into the landscape with chicken wire and growing vines (as Deanna's husband has done). If you can't have a compost heap at home, drop your compost off at a local community garden or subscribe to a compost pickup service.

7. Shop Earth smart

Stay true to your sustainability goals at the store. Even if what goes into your grocery cart is healthy *and* eco-friendly, if it's not needed, it's not sustainable. Similarly, if a new purchase means food at home is wasted, it's not sustainable. We've all impulsively tossed flashy packages (from savvy marketers) into our cart, so that's another reason to steer clear of packaging. Keep a clear head in the store.

Make a list and stick to it. Most of us overbuy when we don't have a list. But sometimes making a meal plan with a corresponding grocery list for *every* meal in the week means we end up with *lots* of groceries, some of which don't get used. In your meal planning, build in days to use up leftovers and make meals from pantry and freezer items.

Bring reusable grocery bags and produce bags to the store. Automatically, put them back in your car after unloading (or have an extra stash) so you always have them on hand. This is especially helpful for spontaneous finds at local roadside stands!

Think about how you can reuse packaging—and pledge to do it when you buy. If you buy it in a package, plan to reuse/recycle/upcycle the package. See guideline #9.

Shop at stores that have bulk aisles. Bring enough bags, jars, and containers to fit all you're buying. Bring a marker for writing the tare weight on your containers, as well as the bulk bin number so you don't have to use a sticker. (Make sure a store allows personal containers by asking at the customer service counter.)

Buy bigger to reduce packaging. Buy the biggest box of crackers instead of two smaller boxes plus their bags. (To keep them from going stale, put in individual containers and keep sealed, or freeze until ready to use; yes, you can freeze crackers!) Buy the largest bag of frozen fruit if you have room in your freezer. Buy two pounds of carrots instead of one pound. Not only will you reduce your use of packaging, but you'll save money too!

8. Conserve while cooking

When we cook, we are using water and energy, which are finite resources. Remember, every little bit helps. Get into the habit of doing some of these things *most* of the time.

Reuse water. Catch the water you use while washing veggies and use it to water your potted herbs. Save pasta cooking water; store in the fridge to reheat leftovers and then use half "saved" and half fresh water the next time you fill a pot to cook pasta. (See our Healthy Kitchen Hack on page 161.)

Boil water quicker. Consider purchasing an electric water kettle (look for used options online at resale sites). You can boil water in about half the time, making your cuppa tea happen faster (and stay hot longer than when microwave-heated). And pasta will be on the table quicker when half or more of the pasta water is heated in the kettle and then transferred to the pot (see the Healthy Kitchen Hack on page 150).

Cut food in smaller pieces. Smaller chunks of chicken and pieces of onion and broccoli will cook quicker. This also helps get dinner done speedily.

Make extra. We have lots of recipes that make extra staples for more than one meal like Speedy Pizza Dough (page 138), Everyday Pot of Lentils (page 170), Savory Sardine Tomato Sauce (page 210), and Spring Chicken with Barley, Carrots, and Artichokes (page 253). Once you get the hang of these, we bet you'll have more ideas on how to batch-cook.

Cover a pot with a lid when cooking. Covering a pot helps keep heat in. Never bring a pot to a boil without covering it first.

Find the right pot. Be sure you're not using a burner that's bigger than your pot or pan—otherwise, that heat gets wasted. For instance, using an 8-inch electric burner to cook something in a 6-inch pot wastes nearly half of the burner's heat, according to EnergyStar.gov.

Use the oven to bake more than one item. After baking something, such as our Spiced Turkish Coffee Coffee Cake (page 39), drizzle some olive oil on whatever veggies you have on hand and roast those in the oven when the cake is done. (Need a recipe for roasted veggies? Try our Honey and Salt Roasted Brussels Sprouts on page 99.)

Get to know how long it takes to heat up your oven. Turn it on *right* before you are ready to use it (instead of before you even start to prep the recipe).

Don't preheat, if possible. It's actually not essential to preheat the oven for casseroles or roasted vegetables (although we specify doing so in this book so our recipes have fewer variables for your success!). For vegetable dishes, casseroles, and meat with cooking times over 30 minutes, simply put the dish in the oven and turn it on. This will take some experimentation, but pretty soon you'll get the hang of what works best and how to adjust specified cooking times. (Note—preheating *is* necessary for baked goods!)

When you *do* preheat, preheat the pan too. In several of our recipes, you will preheat a baking sheet to reduce cooking times and give meat a head start cooking or veggies a crispy "oven-fried" texture when they hit the hot pan.

Microwave first to shorten cooking times. The microwave is extremely energy efficient, reducing cooking energy by up to 80 percent, according to EnergyStar.gov. Just 10 minutes in the microwave can take 40 minutes off baked potatoes (20 to 30 minutes in the oven instead of 60 to 75). Before roasting squash, broccoli, cauliflower, carrots, beets, potato wedges, apples, and other produce, give them a head start in the microwave.

Slow cook what you can. A slow cooker uses the same energy as—or even less than—a light bulb, and we have several slow cooker recipes in this book. Slow cookers, Instant Pots/pressure cookers, and even rice cookers trap heat inside so food cooks without those appliances needing to constantly produce more heat, as in an oven. Use these gadgets more often!

Use the toaster oven. If you have space, or don't have an oven, this appliance can save energy when compared to cooking in a conventional electric oven, almost a 50 percent savings. A toaster oven also offers convection (the same technology used in an air fryer), keeps your kitchen cooler than your traditional oven does in the summer, and is perfect for reheating leftovers.

9. Embrace reusable/recycled food storage and kitchen items

Limit your purchases of store-bought, single-use containers by buying foods in bulk when you can and getting a bit creative with storage items you probably already have in your kitchen. Reusing items helps cut down on energy needed to produce all that packaging, helps decrease the amount of trash you generate, and also helps companies be inspired to reduce some packaging if there is less demand for it.

Go without plastic wrap. If you do have a box of plastic wrap in your kitchen, store it in an inconvenient spot (have a contest with your friends to see how long you can use the same box of plastic wrap; one of us is on three years for the same box!). Use plates or lids to cover dishes in the fridge. Try reusable beeswax wrap.

Use washable towels and napkins. Replacing paper towels and napkins with reusable cloth is probably one of the easiest ways to cut down. Avoid that grocery aisle when you can—remember, our grandmothers managed without them!

Try to avoid buying plastic storage bags. If you must, choose freezer bags, which are sturdier and can be washed and reused again and again. Or reuse the plastic bags that frozen vegetables and fruits come in (which are already engineered to go into the freezer) to freeze your food.

Buy reusable sandwich bags. The designs have come a long way and are even dishwasher safe.

Buy mason jars. They're dishwasher safe and can be used to store foods in the pantry and fridge. Check yard sales and online so you don't have to buy brand-new jars!

Carry around your own cutlery, water bottle, and coffee travel mug. You'll never need another plastic spoon at the ice cream shop. Ask if coffee shops will pour their coffee into your cup.

If you're able to, ditch plastic straws. There are lots of portable—even collapsible—metal and silicone options that you can stash in your car or bag.

Creatively reuse packaging. Use sturdy chip bags for food storage or for lining small garbage bins at home. Reuse pasta sauce, condiment, and glass spice jars for

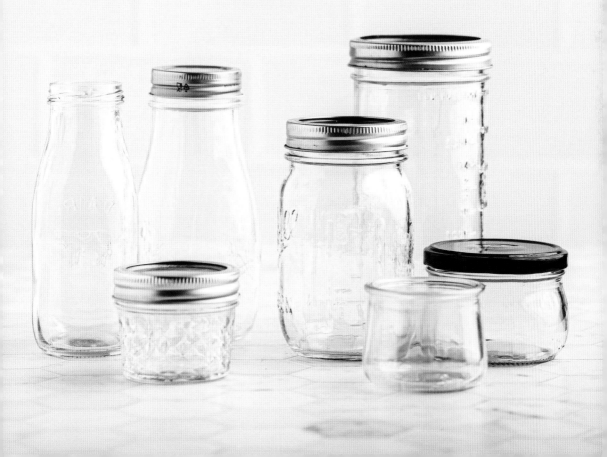

food storage or for sending leftovers home with friends—hummus containers are useful, too. (Deanna even uses jars as vases at home and when gifting flowers!)

Store your leftovers in cracker bags (even liquidy leftovers can be sealed with chip clips or freezer tape). Instead of plastic wrap, place a bowl of leftovers inside a large cereal bag and fold under the opening. And yes, your kids can get used to putting their sandwiches in the plastic bags from dried fruit or frozen vegetables.

10. Support sustainable seafood, meat, and poultry

Since you are reading this book, we bet you've read about how the conventional meat and seafood industries may be contributing to climate change when it comes to greenhouse gas emissions and overfishing. Because it prioritizes veggies and grains, choosing a Mediterranean-style diet is already a step in the right direction! But we believe that seafood, meat, and poultry *can* be part of a sustainable diet; it's all about making smarter choices when you do enjoy these foods.

Making more sustainable choices among these foods gets a bit more complicated, so rather than giving you a quick list, the next two sections are devoted to how you can make more climate-friendly choices.

More Sustainable Seafood

This discussion is complicated because "sustainability" depends on *so* many factors, including fishing practices, species health, population counts, fair labor practices, distances to travel to market, and more. Fishers and aquaculturists are working hard to become more sustainable, so the best guidance on this topic will continue to evolve and change. This section is not intended to be comprehensive; instead, it's a place to begin your journey to eating more sustainable seafood. Search online for current recommendations; we list several certifying organizations on page 18 (like the Marine Stewardship Council).

Navigating the grocery store seafood counter can be intimidating, but your friendly fishmonger can help. And keep in mind that some of the best seafood options come in cans and frozen packages.

Eat a variety. Most Americans usually purchase only four types of seafood: shrimp, salmon, tuna, and cod. Picking a less-popular seafood will mean you're "catching" it before it becomes food waste. If you don't recognize the name, try the fish; ask your fishmonger how to cook it, look at SeafoodNutrition.org, or check our index to see if we have a recipe!

Buy frozen or canned fish. Shockingly, about one-third of all fish caught never gets eaten. This happens for a variety of reasons, but frozen and canned seafood systems are usually the most efficient at getting fish to market. So to help prevent food waste on your watch, gravitate to the freezer or canned fish aisles.

Eat smaller fishes. This might be the *easiest* sustainable seafood: buy canned sardines, herring, mackerel, and anchovies. Being small and lower on the food chain means these fish take less time and ocean resources to reach maturity (often they eat only plankton), and the fish stocks are usually healthier with less chance of being overfished. They are super rich in healthy omega-3 fats and, since they are small, very low in mercury (although that's really not something to worry about with any seafood, since seafood is high in selenium, which offsets any mercury risk). We have lots of recipes for these guys—just a few examples are the Barley, Corn, and Mackerel Medley (page 201), Little Fishes, Red Pepper, and Potato Cakes (page 207), and Zucchini Cavatappi with Invisible Anchovy-Garlic Sauce (page 157). Fun fact: if you like Worcestershire sauce, you already like anchovies, which are an ingredient!

Eat farmed shellfish. The oysters, mussels, clams, and bay scallops available at the fish counter, in the canned seafood aisle, and in the frozen food section are generally raised using environmentally friendly aquaculture practices. They're healthy for you, and these bivalves actually improve the health of the oceans by filtering algae and nutrients from the water, improving the ocean ecosystem.

If you don't live near the coasts, look for local lake fish. Search at the store, but also ask friends who fish locally. Or learn how to fish yourself . . . no matter where you live!

Join a CSF if you live near the ocean. A community-supported fishery program can introduce you to a world of delicious seafood right in your "backyard." Join with a friend—and then learn from the fishers who deliver their catch. LocalCatch.org can help you find a CSF, some of which will ship their catch.

When in doubt, buy US and Canadian (if you reside in North America). Three reasons for this: (1) It's traveled the shortest distance. (2) US and Canadian fishing boats have to follow strict policies to guard against overfishing. (3) These same boats are subject to labor condition requirements that are less transparent on overseas vessels.

Shop smart for shrimp. We won't say never buy shrimp, but it's the most-consumed fish in the US. We don't have a single shrimp recipe in this book because we want to help expand your seafood horizons. When you do buy it, do your research (especially in terms of how far the shrimp has traveled), save shrimp for special occasions (versus everyday), and then be willing to pay the higher price for better shrimp—that money will likely go to getting shrimp back to a more sustainable status.

When traveling, stop at a local fish shop. Buying and cooking local fish is one of the most economical ways to feed a family while traveling. The Ball family has been lucky enough to cook local fish from small fish markets on the Great Lakes and the Florida Gulf to a tiny outdoor market on the coast of South Carolina. At fish shops, get great stories from the fishmongers by asking about how local fish are caught and by whom.

Look for certified seafood. Third-party organizations set high standards for fisheries and supply chain businesses that meet best global practices. Here are the stamps to look for on the seafood you buy:

- Marine Stewardship Council (MSC): one of the easiest logos to find
- Aquaculture Stewardship Council (ASC)
- Global Aquaculture Alliance Best Aquaculture Practices (BAP)
- Canada Organic Aquaculture Standards: for farmed shellfish
- Naturland: for some farmed freshwater fish

More Sustainable Meat and Poultry

You may wonder, Does eating *any* meat fit into a sustainable Mediterranean lifestyle? We did a great deal of research and conducted farmer interviews before we came up with a "yes, but less" answer. While eating less meat is generally the Mediterranean way, in truth, emissions from cattle, including feed production, fuel, and electricity account for just 3.7 percent of total greenhouse gas emission in the US. And if we consume local meat, those transportation emissions are probably less than those for vegetables shipped from across the country. Plus, a more traditional Mediterranean diet pattern does include some poultry and meat. Here are our suggestions:

Enjoy meatless Mondays and Thursdays. You probably won't miss meat if you skip it a few days a week.

Make meat a flavor ingredient instead of a main ingredient. Meat can actually help your family eat more plants—a little animal protein can make vegetables and whole grains more savory and delectable. Many Mediterranean regional cuisines include whole pots of beans flavored with a smaller cut of pork. Vegetable soups and stews are enriched with bits of poultry. Cured beef and pork set out with olives, nuts, and seasonal produce make quick suppers.

Trust and support America's farmers. Today's farms produce the same amount of pork as they did just a few decades ago, but pork producers are doing it on significantly less land, with a quarter less water, and about 10 percent fewer carbon emissions. According to research from animal agriculture across several sectors, greenhouse gas emissions from 1990 to 2005 have remained nearly constant; during the same period total US meat production has increased 50 percent. The future

More Sustainable Seafood Choices

Bay scallops	Buy farmed, and choose fresh, frozen, and/or canned
Canned fish and shellfish	Embraced canned anchovies, clams, herring, mackerel, mussels, oysters, sardines, and trout
Clams	Buy farmed, and choose fresh or canned
Crab	Dungeness crab that's live, fresh, frozen, or canned; almost any variety in cans
Fatty/oily fish	Sustainable varieties include Arctic char, brown trout, rainbow trout, sablefish, Alaskan salmon, and canned salmon with one of the labels from the list on page 18
Mussels	Buy farmed, and choose fresh or canned
Oysters	Buy farmed, and choose fresh or canned
Shrimp	Buy less in general; Oregon pink shrimp (fresh, frozen, or canned), spot prawns from the Pacific Northwest and Alaska, wild shrimp from the US or Canadian North Atlantic, white and pink shrimp from the Gulf of Mexico, USA-farmed shrimp
Tuna	Canned tuna with one of the labels from the list on page 18
White fish	Sustainable choices include pollock, hake from Europe, silver hake, Atlantic whiting, flounder, barramundi, some haddock/scrod

looks even brighter as members of the North American Meat Institute have pledged ambitious goals for animal care, food safety, labor and human rights, and health and wellness. Support American farmers moving to change a giant industry that is now working hard to meet consumer demand for sustainable meat—at the same time that consumers still expect inexpensive meat. Be willing to pay more for your meat as farmers make these changes.

Read sustainability statements. Large brand-name meat production/processing companies list their statements on their websites. Do your homework. When you do, you may find that some companies are doing more than others.

Help farmers feed the world. By 2050, the world will have to find a way to feed an additional 2 billion people, according to some estimates. Today, each American farmer feeds about 144 people worldwide. Meat is a high-quality protein to nourish urban populations. US ranchers generally graze cows on arid scrubland that is not productive for producing plant crops. Grazing animals on this land more than *doubles* the area that can be used to produce food in the US. Cattle and sheep ranchers upcycle the plants from rocky, steep lands into nutrient-rich meat.

Celebrate the soil. Farmers and ranchers list soil as their number one asset. So rotating crops and grazing animals, protecting water sources, reducing chemical use, and planting lentils and sunflower seeds and other soil-enriching crops are their most important farming tools. If you join a local meat share—which is also a very smart choice—ask your farmer if you can support their other farming efforts by purchasing some of the farm's other crops that help with soil enrichment.

Eat local meat. Not only will you cut down on miles the meat travels, but you'll be supporting healthy soil at a farm near you. To find local meat sources, start at farmers' markets; these locals may even offer meat share programs to help you and a few friends split the meat of a whole animal. Not only is it fun to get to know some local farmers, but it's also a great way to help families learn to use every part of an animal.

Eat underused cuts. Remember, a pig has only two tenderloins, and a chicken has only two drumsticks. So if you purchase the same cuts of meat over and over again, it's not the most sustainable way to shop. Luckily, the less popular cuts are also some of the most budget-friendly, as we list in the following "More Sustainable Meat and Poultry Choices" table. If you have access, start at your local butcher shop that breaks down whole animals; ask what some of the least popular cuts are, especially since cuts are known by unique names in different parts of the country. (See our recipe for Cumin-Marinated Steak with Charred Peppers and Onions on page 236 and a recipe for cooking a whole chicken on page 253.)

More Sustainable Meat and Poultry Choices

Beef	Ground beef; charcoal, oyster, Denver, sirloin flap, coulotte, and merlot steaks; brisket flat half; stew meat; chuck eye roast; cross rib roast
Lamb	Anything *but* lamb chops and leg of lamb
Pork	Ground pork, pork skirt steak, sirloin chops, pork collar, pork shoulder, pork loin roast
Chicken and Turkey	Whole birds

Use It or Lose It

Here are a few ideas for what to do with leftover ingredients and meals to avoid food waste.

Part of an onion
- Make quick pickled onions (page 134).
- Drizzle with olive oil and roast when the oven is already on for something else.

Chickpea liquid from a can
- Add to canned or homemade soups to thicken and add extra B vitamins.
- Use in baking as an egg substitute.

Leftover cooked or canned beans
- Mash and add to ground meat to extend it.
- Mash, add extra bean liquid, and puree. Put an egg on it for breakfast or dinner.
- Add to any whole grain—even unsweetened oatmeal—for lunch.

Canned tomatoes
- Cook an egg in them; add herbs.
- Serve over barley, farro, or pasta; add any canned seafood.
- Make our Very Veggie Sustainable Soup for One (page 111).

Canned pumpkin
- Whisk into vegetable- or tomato-based soup, chili, or pasta sauce.
- Mix into cooked or overnight oats.

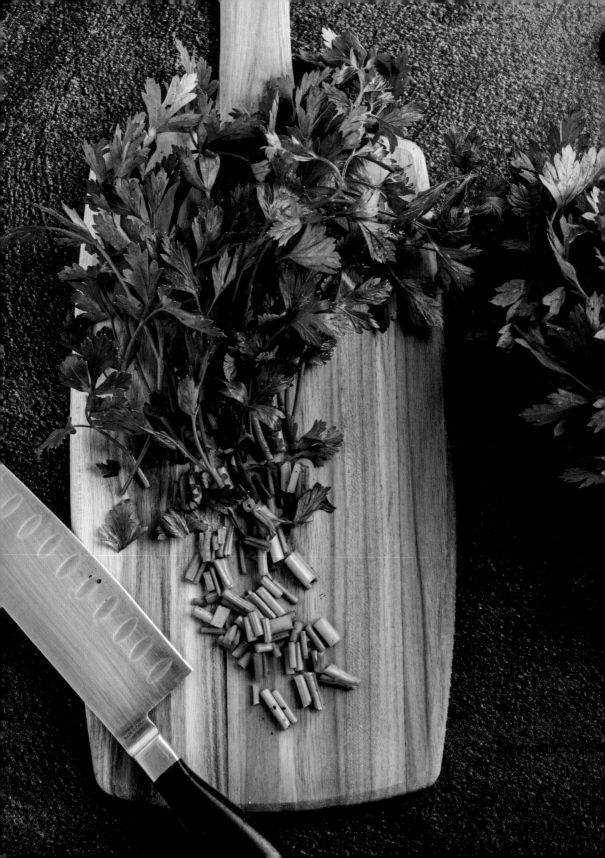

Lemon juice
- Make a buttermilk substitute for baking: Put 1 tablespoon lemon juice in a measuring cup and add milk up to the 1-cup line for 1 cup "buttermilk."
- Freeze juice in ice cube trays to throw into soup, stews, salad dressings, or baked goods.

Lemon zest
- Add to pancakes, muffins, and oatmeal.
- Make DIY Za'atar spice: grated lemon zest + dried thyme + toasted sesame seeds + salt.

Whole grains including farro, bulgur, barley, oatmeal
- Eat as a savory breakfast topped with za'atar and olive oil or cheese.
- Add to ground meat to extend for burgers, meatloaf, or meatballs.

Berries that are starting to droop
- Blend into smoothies or salad dressings.
- Freeze and use as an "ice cube" to flavor water.

Pasta cooking water
- Before it cools, poach a few eggs in it. Then refrigerate the eggs for quick meals.
- Store in the fridge for warming up leftover stews and casseroles; the starchy water helps improve the texture.

Veggie scraps like peels and trimmings
- Make Veggie Scraps Broth (page 120).

Leftover herbs, like cilantro, parsley, basil, mint—both leaves and tender stems
- Use by the cupful in any recipe that calls for just a tablespoon or two.
- Add to any green salad.
- Toss into scrambled eggs, pasta sauce, soups, and stews.

Liquid from jarred or canned veggies, like mushrooms and roasted red peppers
- Add to Veggie Scraps Broth (page 120).
- Thin out pesto, as in Cauliflower Steaks with Sun-Dried Tomato and Basil Pesto (page 175).
- Add to soups.

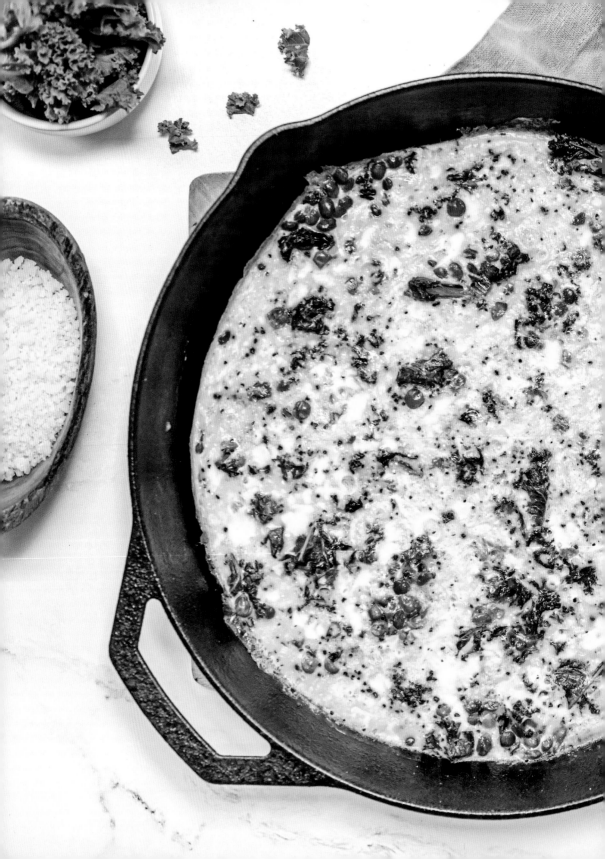

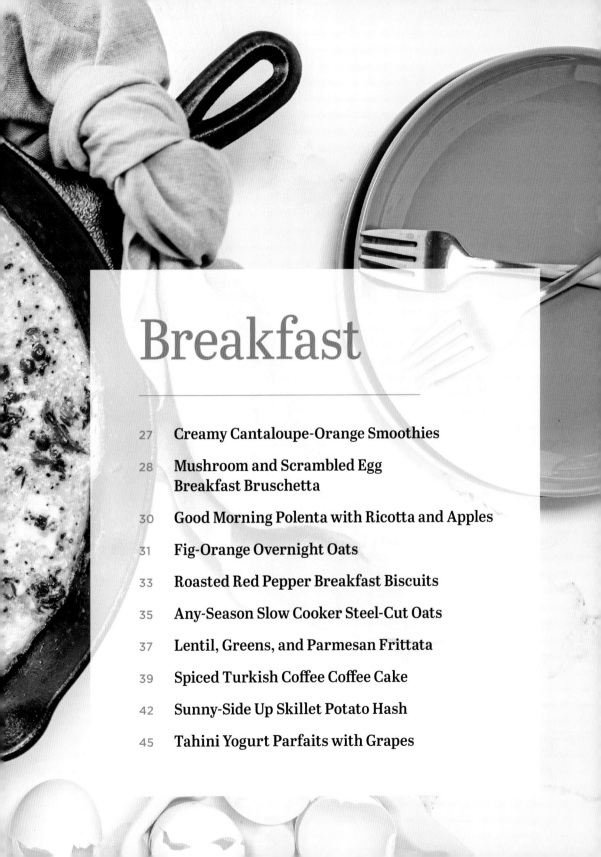

Breakfast

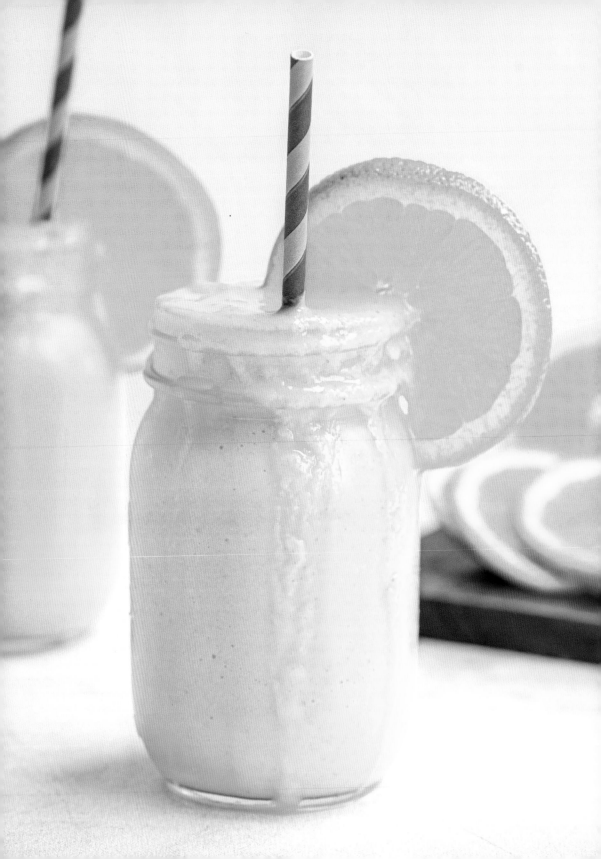

Creamy Cantaloupe-Orange Smoothies

SERVES 2
Prep time: 5 minutes

1 mandarin orange, unpeeled, quartered, *or* half a navel orange

⅔ cup plain whole-milk Greek yogurt

½ cup 2% milk

½ teaspoon vanilla extract

2 tablespoons honey

2½ cups cubed cantaloupe, frozen

4 ice cubes

Did you know you can eat the entire orange, peel and all? Tossing the whole fruit in the blender has many benefits: It gives you the nutrition from the peel, which contains fiber, potent antioxidants, and nearly three times more vitamin C than the inner fruit. It cuts down on food waste. And, most importantly, it imparts the most luscious orange flavor! Not only will this sunny Mediterranean fruit smoothie wake up your taste buds, but it also takes virtually no time to make since there's no need to peel the orange and you can freeze the cantaloupe the night before. Alas, cantaloupe rinds are not edible, so compost those but save the seeds (see our Healthy Kitchen Hack on page 261)!

Puree the orange, yogurt, milk, and vanilla in a blender until smooth. With the blender running, remove the center opening of the blender lid and drizzle in the honey, then drop in the cantaloupe pieces and ice cubes one at a time. Blend until smooth. Divide between 2 glasses and serve immediately.

Healthy Kitchen Hack: To pick the perfect cantaloupe, honeydew, or other round melon, sniff the ends. Select a melon with a strong, sweet melon aroma. Watermelon is a bit different; look for a watermelon that's heavy for its size and has a light yellow spot where the fruit sat on the ground and ripened.

"My boys and I liked this with frozen blueberries, too. It's fun to throw a whole mandarin orange in!"

—April from Pendleton, OR

Per Serving: Calories: 312; Total Fat: 6g; Saturated Fat: 3g; Cholesterol: 16mg; Sodium: 94mg; Total Carbohydrates: 56g; Fiber: 6g; Protein: 13g

Mushroom and Scrambled Egg Breakfast Bruschetta

SERVES 4

Prep time: 10 minutes
Cook time: 15 minutes

2 tablespoons extra-virgin olive oil, divided

2 cups sliced mushrooms (8 ounces), any variety

6 large eggs

½ teaspoon kosher or sea salt

¼ teaspoon black pepper

⅓ cup chopped fresh herbs of choice, leaves and stems, plus more for garnish if desired

1 garlic clove, cut in half

8 (¾-inch-thick) slices baguette-style whole-grain bread *or* 4 slices larger Italian-style whole-grain bread, toasted

You've never tasted the classic combo of eggs and toast like this before! These scrambled eggs are luscious thanks to an extra swirl of extra-virgin olive oil. Ditto for the mushrooms—the trick to hearty, flavorful mushrooms (especially specialty varieties—see the Hack) is to also cook them in EVOO. With the protein-packed eggs and the fiber-filled mushrooms, this yummy dish will keep you satisfied until lunch while delivering some fresh greens to start your day—we like using dill, cilantro, parsley, basil, or a combination of whatever we have on hand.

In a large skillet over medium heat, heat 1 tablespoon oil. Add the mushrooms and cook until most of the mushroom liquid has evaporated, about 8 minutes, stirring occasionally.

While the mushrooms cook, in a small bowl, whisk together the eggs, 2 tablespoons water, the salt, and the pepper. Mix in the herbs.

Turn the heat down to medium-low. Push the mushrooms to the outer edges of the skillet. Add the remaining 1 tablespoon oil and swirl it around the pan. Pour the egg mixture into the skillet. Stir in the mushrooms and cook until the eggs are soft-scrambled, 3 to 5 minutes, stirring occasionally. Remove from the heat.

Rub one side of each piece of toast with the cut side of the garlic clove halves. (Save the garlic for another recipe.) Spoon the egg mixture on top of each piece of toast, garnish with additional herbs if desired, and serve.

Healthy Kitchen Hack: While this breakfast is delish with regular white button mushrooms, if you happen to get your hands on locally grown or wild mushrooms, it will likely be even better. Most areas of the country now have regional mushroom growers, so you can get gorgeous shiitakes, oyster mushrooms, or morels at farmers' markets, in CSAs, or from foragers (those who gather wild mushrooms). If you get the chance, learn how to hunt for mushrooms safely from a professional forager to better appreciate all the bounty growing wild near you—Serena forages every spring for morels near where she lives in rural Southern Illinois.

Per Serving: **Calories: 252; Total Fat: 14g; Saturated Fat: 3g; Cholesterol: 279mg; Sodium: 452mg; Total Carbohydrates: 17g; Fiber: 1g; Protein: 11g**

Good Morning Polenta with Ricotta and Apples

SERVES 4
Prep time: 10 minutes
Cook time: 15 minutes

2 cups 2% milk

¼ teaspoon kosher or sea salt

1 cup yellow cornmeal

1 batch Made-in-Minutes Homemade Ricotta Cheese (page 48) *or* ¾ cup store-bought whole-milk ricotta cheese

1 tablespoon honey, divided

1 teaspoon ground cinnamon, divided

2 apples, cored and sliced

If you want a speedy hot breakfast beyond your usual bowl of oatmeal, keep a bag of cornmeal, polenta, or corn grits in your pantry—all are variations of ground corn. We like the stone-ground whole corn versions, which are whole grains and have a coarser texture. Here, creamy ricotta and sweet, cinnamon-dusted apples make for some delectable mix-ins for your hot grain morning meal. And much like oatmeal, morning polenta can be jazzed up in so many ways—look to this recipe's Healthy Kitchen Hack for some additional corn porridge inspiration!

In a medium stockpot, pour in the milk along with 1½ cups water. Add the salt and bring to a boil over medium-high heat. Reduce the heat to medium, then slowly pour in the cornmeal, whisking constantly for about 1 minute. Reduce the heat to medium-low and continue to cook the polenta until thickened, stirring frequently, 6 to 8 minutes (the polenta will be thick). Remove from the heat and let cool for about 5 minutes.

Slowly whisk in the ricotta, 2 teaspoons honey, and ½ teaspoon cinnamon. Divide into four cereal bowls and top with sliced apples. Divide and drizzle the remaining 1 teaspoon honey and sprinkle the remaining ½ teaspoon cinnamon over each bowl of breakfast polenta.

Healthy Kitchen Hack: For some yummy and sustainable variations of this dish, swap in fresh seasonal fruit for the apples, like pears in the winter and fresh peaches in the summer. Or rely on your stash of frozen fruit, like frozen berries or frozen mango chunks, any time of year. Stir in at the end of cooking, and the residual heat will thaw the fruit. For an extra protein punch, sprinkle on a tablespoon per serving of your favorite chopped nuts (and be sure to store those nuts in the freezer to extend their shelf life).

Per Serving: Calories: 317; Total Fat: 10g; Saturated Fat: 6g; Cholesterol: 34mg; Sodium: 229mg; Total Carbohydrates: 48g; Fiber: 5g; Protein: 12g

Fig-Orange Overnight Oats

SERVES 4
Prep time: 10 minutes
Chill time: Overnight

1⅓ cups gluten-free old-fashioned rolled oats

1 (11-ounce) can mandarin oranges in juice, drained, *or* 1 large orange, peeled and chopped
Save the juice—see the Hack

½ cup chopped pecans

¼ cup chopped dried figs *or* 3 large fresh figs, chopped

1 tablespoon honey

¼ teaspoon freshly grated nutmeg or ground nutmeg

¼ teaspoon kosher or sea salt

1 cup plain 2% Greek yogurt

¾ cup 2% milk

Overnight oats are one of our top sustainable breakfasts as there's no energy for cooking required. What's more, oats are an important part of crop rotation, a sustainable farming strategy to keep the soil rich and diverse (not to mention you can buy them in large containers or even in bulk to cut back on packaging waste). The fig-orange combo here is classically Mediterranean, and to be more eco-friendly, we use dried figs and canned mandarin oranges—but you can certainly use the fresh versions when they're in season!

In a large container that has a lid, mix together the oats, oranges, pecans, figs, honey, nutmeg, and salt. Add the yogurt and milk and mix until everything is well incorporated. Cover and refrigerate overnight (or for at least 8 hours).

To serve, divide into four bowls or to-go containers.

Healthy Kitchen Hack: Go full-on Mediterranean and drizzle a little bit of olive oil and an extra pinch of salt over your overnight oats when serving! It might sound strange, but the buttery olive oil and salt pair deliciously with the sweet and nutty flavors. Also, when you buy canned or jarred fruit that's packed in juice, don't just dump the liquid when you've used the fruit. You can drink the juice or mix it with seltzer for a refreshing beverage—and you can even add some of your favorite spirit for a fruity cocktail!

Per Serving: Calories: 327; Total Fat: 12g; Saturated Fat: 3g; Cholesterol: 9mg; Sodium: 123mg; Total Carbohydrates: 42g; Fiber: 6g; Protein: 13g

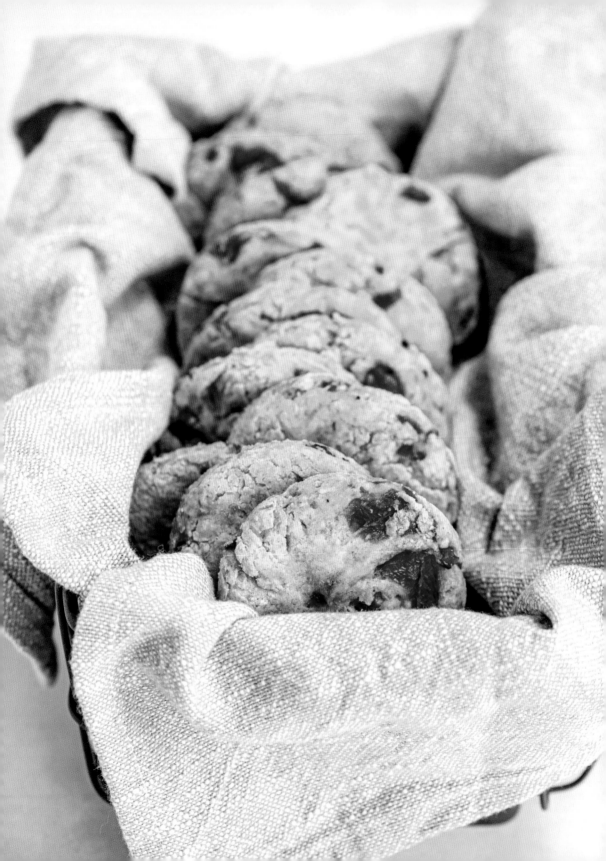

Roasted Red Pepper Breakfast Biscuits

MAKES 10 BISCUITS (SERVES 10)
Prep time: 15 minutes
Cook time: 20 minutes

¼ **cup jarred diced roasted red peppers**
Save the remaining peppers and liquid for another recipe

1 **cup whole-wheat flour, plus more for dusting**

1 **cup all-purpose flour**

2 **teaspoons baking powder**

½ **teaspoon kosher or sea salt**

¼ **cup extra-virgin olive oil**

⅔ **cup plain whole-milk Greek yogurt**

To us, brunch means we slow down to enjoy the food along with our family or company; that's the Mediterranean way! And these hearty, add-what-you-wish biscuits are perfect for a leisurely mid-morning meal. We mixed in roasted red peppers, but feel free to add ingredients you need to use up, like fresh herbs, raisins, or crumbled cheese. Or go a step further and turn them into upscale breakfast sandwiches using the super easy, baked eggs technique in our Hack. The assembled breakfast sandwiches freeze beautifully, making them ideal for hurried weekday mornings.

Preheat the oven to 400°F. Spread a sheet of parchment paper on a large rimmed baking sheet.

Arrange the diced peppers on a clean kitchen towel to absorb extra moisture.

In a large bowl, whisk together the whole-wheat flour, all-purpose flour, baking powder, and salt. With a fork, stir in the oil until the dough is crumbly. Add the yogurt and stir (not all the flour will be incorporated). Sprinkle a little whole-wheat flour on the counter and dump out the biscuit dough; sprinkle the red peppers over the dough. Knead the dough just until all the ingredients are incorporated (about 25 times); the dough will be crumbly. Gently press and shape the dough into a 9-inch square. Using a 3-inch metal canning ring or the rim of a drinking glass, cut out nine biscuits; press the remaining scraps together and free-form shape into one more biscuit. Arrange the biscuits on the lined baking sheet, about 1 inch apart.

Bake for 18 to 20 minutes, until the biscuits just begin to turn slightly golden. Do not overbake. Serve with the baked eggs below if desired.

Healthy Kitchen Hack: Since your oven is already on to make these biscuits, in about 15 minutes, you can have

continued

Roasted Red Pepper Breakfast Biscuits *(continued)*

custardy baked eggs to make breakfast sammies! Here's how to make sandwich-friendly eggs in a sheet pan:

After baking the biscuits, lower the oven temp to 300°F. Brush a large rimmed baking sheet with 1½ teaspoons olive oil.

In a bowl, whisk together 12 eggs, ¼ cup 2% milk, ½ teaspoon kosher or sea salt, and ¼ cup chopped fresh herbs or spinach (optional).

Pour onto the prepared baking sheet and bake for 15 minutes or until the eggs are just set. Cool slightly and cut into 10 rectangles.

To make a sandwich, cut a biscuit in half, fold over the egg rectangle to fit, and lay it on the cut biscuit half. Top with the remaining biscuit half. Serve right way, or wrap the assembled sandwiches in aluminum foil and store in the freezer. To serve, heat the wrapped frozen sandwich in a toaster oven until warm, 10 to 15 minutes.

Per Serving (1 biscuit): **Calories: 155; Total Fat: 7g; Saturated Fat: 1g; Cholesterol: 2mg; Sodium: 115mg; Total Carbohydrates: 20g; Fiber: 2g; Protein: 5g**

Per Serving (1 biscuit plus egg filling): **Calories: 249; Total Fat: 13g; Saturated Fat: 3g; Cholesterol: 225mg; Sodium: 289mg; Total Carbohydrates: 22g; Fiber: 2g; Protein: 12g**

Any-Season Slow Cooker Steel-Cut Oats

SERVES 6
Prep time: 10 minutes
Cook time: 4 to 8 hours

1 tablespoon extra-virgin olive oil

2 cups 2% milk

1½ cups gluten-free steel-cut oats

1 cup unsweetened applesauce

1 tablespoon vanilla extract

1½ teaspoons ground cinnamon

½ teaspoon ground cardamom (optional)

¼ teaspoon kosher or sea salt

3 cups chopped fresh or frozen fruit *or* ¾ cups chopped dried fruit

⅓ cup seeds or nuts of choice, tahini, or nut butter

We love our eco-friendly slow cookers (did we mention that it uses only as much energy as a light bulb?). Steel-cut oats hold up well in a slow cooker, while old-fashioned oats tend to turn very soft. And oats are a perfect palette to experiment with combinations of mix-ins from all the shelf-stable goodies in your pantry—like nut butter, nuts, or seeds (think pumpkin, sunflower, or sesame)—and frozen fruit in your freezer. But also feel free to toss in any seasonal fresh fruit you may have on hand, especially produce that needs to be "saved" from the back of the refrigerator. If you need some inspiration, start with one of our favorite Mediterranean combinations of dried apricots, pistachios, and tahini.

Pour the oil into a 4- to 7-quart slow cooker. Brush the oil all over the inside of the cooker and then also coat with cooking spray. (The oats will stick to the inside if not well oiled.) In the slow cooker, stir together 4½ cups water, the milk, oats, applesauce, vanilla, cinnamon, cardamom (if using), and salt. Cover and cook on low for 7 to 8 hours (start before bedtime if you get up early) or on high for 4 hours, until the oats are soft but still a bit chewy. Stir well and then mix in or top with your favorite fruits, seeds, and/or nuts.

Note: Turn the slow cooker off or to the warm setting right after the cooking time is up; otherwise, the oats will become crusty and may burn.

Healthy Kitchen Hack: In a 7-quart or larger slow cooker, double this recipe to get you and your family through the week or freeze the extras for future meals. Portion into individual containers and store in the freezer for up to 4 months. Frozen portions can be reheated in the microwave for a quick breakfast or even a last-minute lunch or light dinner!

Per Serving (with dried apricots, pistachios, and tahini): Calories: 366; Total Fat: 14g; Saturated Fat: 3g; Cholesterol: 7mg; Sodium: 137mg; Total Carbohydrates: 51g; Fiber: 6g; Protein: 11g

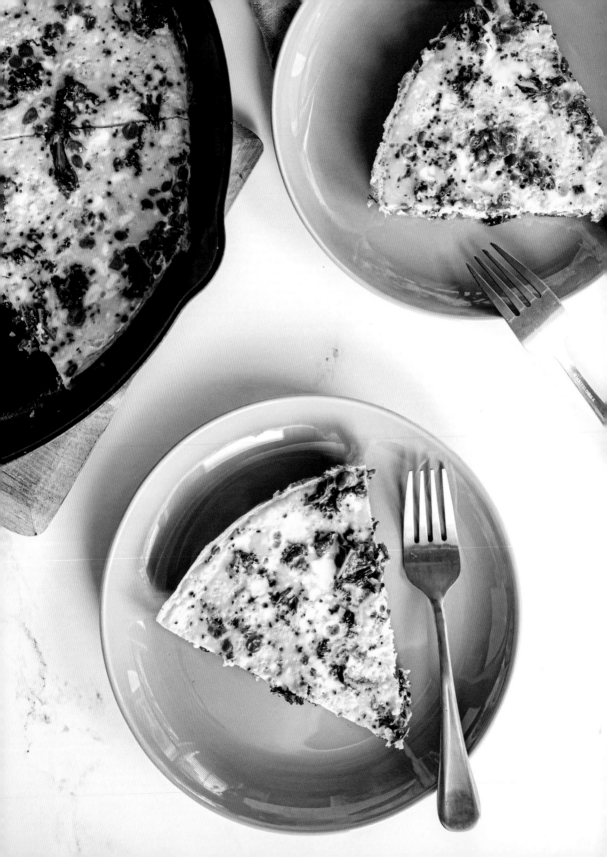

Lentil, Greens, and Parmesan Frittata

SERVES 6
Prep time: 10 minutes
Cook time: 35 minutes

2 tablespoons extra-virgin olive oil, divided

6 scallions (green onions), green and white parts, thinly sliced
Save the stem roots! See page 70

1 teaspoon ground cumin

4 cups chopped dark leafy greens

7 large eggs

¼ cup 2% milk

½ teaspoon kosher or sea salt

¼ teaspoon black pepper

1½ cups cooked brown lentils (see page 170) *or* **1 (15-ounce) can lentils, drained and rinsed**
Save the liquid for another use

¾ cup grated Parmesan cheese

Protein- and plant-packed, this filling frittata will power you through your morning, but don't write it off as just a breakfast dish; it works for any mealtime—served hot or cold. This recipe will also get you into more eco-friendly habits, like using up any leafy greens like kale, Swiss chard, spinach, mustard greens, collards, and fresh herbs that you might have lurking in your fridge, and leaning on lentils more prominently in your cooking routine (see the Healthy Kitchen Hack). Lastly, this frittata cooks solely on your stovetop versus the more traditional method of cooking both on a burner and in the oven, reducing the cooking energy needed. We also "skipped the flip," so there's no last-minute stress with trying to get the frittata out of the skillet without a mishap!

In a 12-inch skillet (cast iron works best) over medium heat, heat 1 tablespoon oil. Add the scallions and cumin and cook for 1 minute, stirring frequently. Add the greens and cook for another 3 to 5 minutes, until wilted, stirring occasionally.

While the greens cook, in a medium bowl, whisk together the eggs, milk, salt, and pepper. Set aside.

Once the greens are wilted, push them to the side of the pan, add the remaining 1 tablespoon oil, and swirl it around the pan. Add the lentils and Parmesan cheese, stirring a few times to combine with the greens. Pour the egg mixture over the top and tilt the skillet until the egg evenly covers the lentils. Cook until the edges start to set, 1 to 2 minutes.

Cover the skillet with a lid or a large rimmed baking sheet, turn the heat to medium-low, and cook for 15 minutes. Uncover and check the center. If it's still runny, cover again and cook for another 5 minutes. Once the center is just about set, remove from the stove and let sit, covered, for another 5 minutes to complete the cooking process and let the frittata begin to pull away from the edges of the skillet (the bottom will have a

continued

slight crust from the lentils and cheese). Cut into 6 wedges and serve warm or at room temperature. Refrigerate (or freeze) any leftovers—the frittata wedges are also delicious cold and make for a great grab-and-go breakfast or an instant sandwich filling.

Healthy Kitchen Hack: A type of pulse, super affordable lentils have one of the lowest carbon footprints of all crops *and* they're rich in protein, which are just a few reasons we love having them in our cooking routine. If you can't find canned lentils, cook up a double batch following our Everyday Pot of Lentils recipe (page 170). Drain, cool, and store in reusable freezer bags for up to 5 days in the refrigerator or 6 months in the freezer.

Per Serving: Calories: 260; Total Fat: 14g; Saturated Fat: 5g; Cholesterol: 229mg; Sodium: 478mg; Total Carbohydrates: 17g; Fiber: 5g; Protein: 16g

"This was easy to make—I liked that it didn't use a lot of dishes and that it's heart-healthy! Would also be a great side dish with breakfast meats."

—**Christine from Bryn Mawr, PA**

Spiced Turkish Coffee Coffee Cake

SERVES 12
Prep time: 10 minutes
Cook time: 35 minutes

3 cups gluten-free old-fashioned or quick oats, divided

½ cup chopped walnuts, pecans, or almonds

4 tablespoons extra-virgin olive oil, divided

¾ cup sugar, divided

1 teaspoon ground cinnamon

½ teaspoon ground cardamom

½ teaspoon ground nutmeg

⅜ teaspoon kosher or sea salt, divided

2 teaspoons baking powder

¾ cup plain whole-milk Greek yogurt

½ cup very strong coffee, room temperature or cooled, or cold brew

Or, swap in 1½ teaspoons instant coffee mixed with ½ cup water

3 large eggs

1½ teaspoons vanilla extract

Nope, the title isn't a typo! This is really a double-coffee cake because it goes great with coffee and has coffee baked right in. While true Turkish coffee is made by a precise stovetop method, one cup at a time, many of us start our day slightly more rushed, making a pot of coffee or grabbing a cold brew instead. This reality often means leftover coffee. Use it to make this "yes, you can have cake for breakfast" coffee cake (Serena's son was thrilled with that idea!). Made with a base of whole-grain oat flour, the batter comes together quickly in the blender, bakes into a hearty cake texture, and boasts the same amount of fiber and even more protein than a bowl of oatmeal. And we think you'll agree that the cinnamon sugar–Turkish spiced topping is the proverbial icing on this filling breakfast cake.

Preheat the oven to 350°F. Coat a 9-inch square baking dish or pan with cooking spray.

For the crumble topping, in a medium bowl, mix together ½ cup oats, the nuts, 2 tablespoons oil, 2 tablespoons sugar, the cinnamon, cardamom, nutmeg, and ⅛ teaspoon salt and set aside.

For the cake batter, process the remaining 2½ cups oats in a blender or food processor until they become a fine flour. Add the baking powder and remaining ¼ teaspoon salt; pulse once or twice to combine. Add the remaining 2 tablespoons oil, remaining ½ cup + 2 tablespoons sugar, yogurt, coffee, eggs, and vanilla and blend until smooth (the batter will be thin). Pour into the prepared pan.

Bake for 15 minutes. Carefully remove the hot baking dish and sprinkle on the crumble topping. Return to the oven and bake for an additional 12 minutes (for a glass or ceramic dish) to 15 minutes (for a metal pan), until the topping is crisp and the cake springs back when pressed in the center. Serve warm or at room temperature.

Healthy Kitchen Hack: Don't dump that little bit of coffee left in the pot! Have a "coffee jar" in your fridge to save leftover coffee. Besides making this breakfast cake, you

continued

Spiced Turkish Coffee Coffee Cake *(continued)*

can mix it with milk and cook oatmeal in it, freeze it in ice cube trays for iced coffee, use it to add a contrasting bitterness to chili or meat stews, pour it over vanilla yogurt or ice cream, or dilute it and then use it to water your acid-loving plants.

Per Serving: Calories: 228; Total Fat: 9g; Saturated Fat: 2g; Cholesterol: 48mg; Sodium: 104mg; Total Carbohydrates: 29g; Fiber: 3g; Protein: 7g

"My whole family loved the dense, moist texture. Our kids thought it tasted a bit like their favorite baked oatmeal. The blender method was so easy that even my 4-year-old could make it."

—Dawn from Hamel, IL

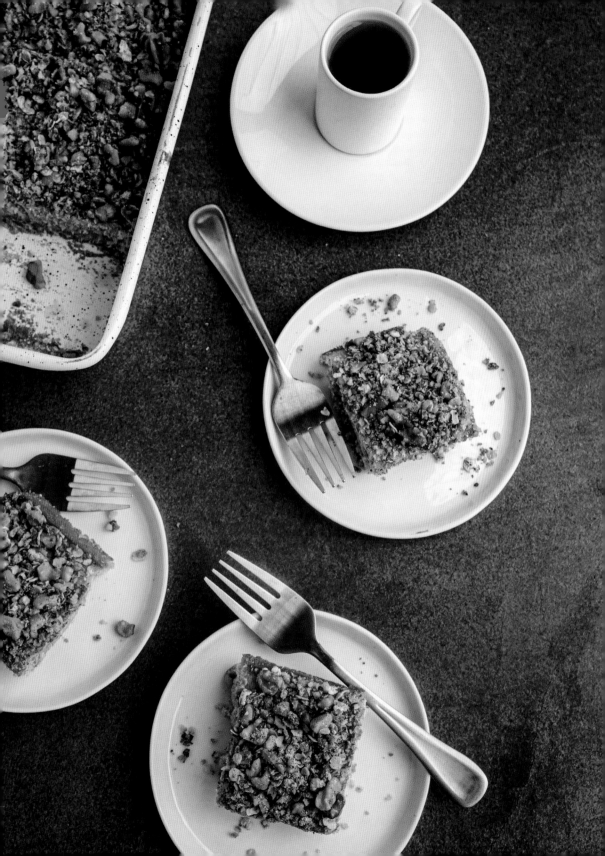

Sunny-Side Up Skillet Potato Hash

SERVES 4

Prep time: 10 minutes
Cook time: 15 minutes

3 tablespoons extra-virgin olive oil, divided

1 medium onion (any type), chopped

1 sweet bell pepper (any color), seeded and chopped

4 cups frozen shredded hash brown potatoes

½ teaspoon kosher or sea salt

1½ cups chopped fresh tomatoes or undrained canned diced tomatoes

1 tablespoon red wine vinegar

4 large eggs

1 cup chopped fresh cilantro or parsley, leaves and stems

Several hours later, the compliments came for this dish from Serena's father. Farmer Bob is a man of few words. And brunch in the Ball household, with five kids, is a very loud occasion, so sometimes it's hard to get a word in edgewise. But these gussied-up hash browns made such an impression on Bob that later that evening he said, "Those skillet potatoes today were really, really good." We think you'll also get rave reviews for this fresh take on hash browns using one of our favorite simple meal-solution ingredients: a big bag of last-in-the-freezer-for-months, no-waste, frozen shredded potatoes. Make your hash more Mediterranean by mixing ½ teaspoon smoked paprika, za'atar, or thyme with the salt.

In a large cast iron or nonstick skillet over medium heat, heat 2 tablespoons oil. Add the onion and bell pepper and cook, stirring occasionally, until they just start to soften, about 5 minutes. Using a spatula, push the vegetables to the outer edges of the skillet. Pour in the remaining 1 tablespoon oil and swirl it around the pan. When the oil has heated, spread the frozen potatoes evenly in the pan. Sprinkle with the salt and cover with a lid (or a baking sheet if you don't have a lid). Cook, without stirring, until the potatoes begin to turn golden brown, about 5 minutes. Then continue to cook, stirring occasionally, until most of the potatoes are golden brown, an additional 3 to 5 minutes. Add the tomatoes and vinegar and cook, stirring and scraping up any browned bits, for about 2 more minutes. Evenly smooth out the mixture in the skillet.

Using the back of a large spoon, make four hollowed-out areas in the vegetable mixture. Working quickly, crack an egg into a small bowl or cup and then carefully pour it into one of the indentations. Repeat the process with the remaining 3 eggs. Cover the skillet and cook until the whites are set but the yolks are still runny, 5 to 8 minutes. (Some of the potatoes will be crispy but more will be softer, but all will have a yummy toasted flavor.) Top with the cilantro and serve immediately.

Healthy Kitchen Hack: What to do with the rest of that bag of frozen hash browns? Here's one idea: Follow the package instructions for cooking half the bag (about 6 cups) on the stovetop with 1 to 2 tablespoons extra-virgin olive oil and ½ teaspoon salt. Top with canned beans, fresh herbs, and hot sauce (or other favorite condiment in your fridge). Or layer with mozzarella cheese, roasted red peppers, and sliced olives and drizzle with tomato sauce for a potato-crust pizza. For Greek-style hash brown potatoes, turn to page 64 for topping ideas from our Loaded Greek Potato Chips.

Per Serving: Calories: 377; Total Fat: 17g; Saturated Fat: 4g; Cholesterol: 186mg; Sodium: 371mg; Total Carbohydrates: 46g; Fiber: 6g; Protein: 12g

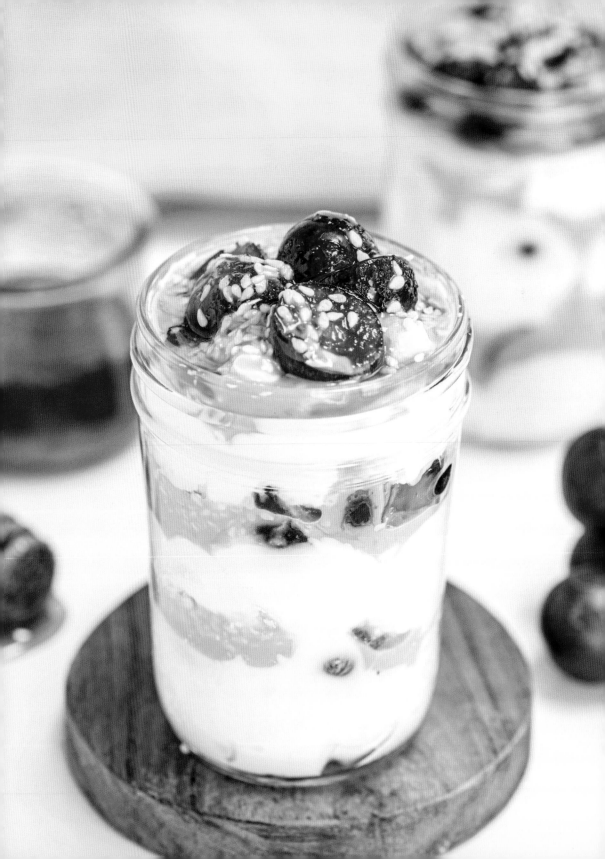

Tahini Yogurt Parfaits with Grapes

SERVES 2
Prep time: 10 minutes

1½ cups vanilla
2% Greek yogurt,
divided

2 tablespoons tahini,
divided

1½ cups halved
seedless grapes
(about 50 whole
grapes)

1 tablespoon sesame
seeds, divided

1 teaspoon honey,
divided

Here's our Mediterranean version of the American classic combo of PB&J . . . but for breakfast. Tahini—the drizzle-able sesame seed paste that's a Middle Eastern staple—makes for a delish and slightly different flavor swap for peanut butter. And of course, fresh grapes are a more wholesome and nutritious counterpart to jelly! Feel free to also use different berries when in season, and if you'd prefer to reduce the sweetness, use plain Greek yogurt instead of vanilla flavored.

To assemble the parfaits, spoon ¼ cup yogurt into the bottom of two tall glasses. Spoon 1 teaspoon of tahini into each parfait and top each with ¼ cup cut grapes. Sprinkle each with ½ teaspoon sesame seeds and then repeat the layering process two more times. Drizzle the top of each parfait with ½ teaspoon honey and serve.

Healthy Kitchen Hack: One of our recipe pet peeves is calling for an obscure ingredient that you then stow away in your pantry, spice drawer, or refrigerator, never to be seen again until it's tossed out. If you are new to tahini, we want to encourage you to make it an item you reach for more often. Along with trading it for nut butter in just about any recipe, try it whisked into plain Greek yogurt with honey for an enticing spread/dip/dressing. Or, use it to make a speedy homemade hummus like our Pumpkin Hummus on page 63 or our Lemon Hummus on page 231. Mix it into your hot grain breakfast cereal or spread it over waffles and pancakes topped with fruit and a drizzle of honey. And for an easy, delectable homemade dessert, whip up our Chocolate Tahini Pudding Cups on page 273.

Per Serving: Calories: 308; Total Fat: 11g; Saturated Fat: 2g; Cholesterol: 3mg; Sodium: 47mg; Total Carbohydrates: 44g; Fiber: 3g; Protein: 14g

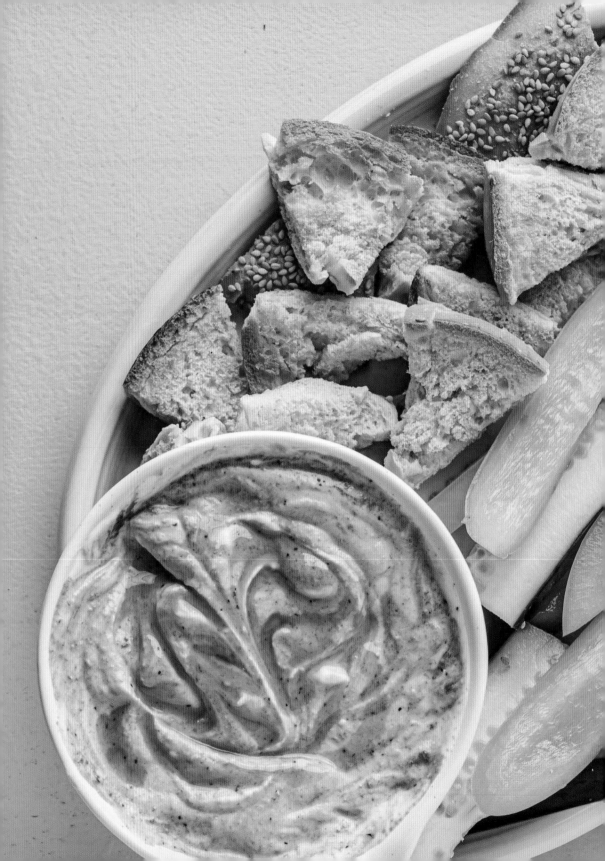

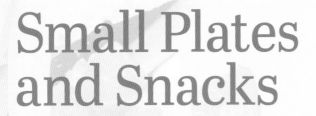

Small Plates and Snacks

Made-in-Minutes Homemade Ricotta Cheese

MAKES ABOUT ¾ CUP (SERVES 6)
Prep time: 10 minutes
Cook time: 10 minutes

4 cups whole or 2% milk

1 cup buttermilk or plain kefir

⅛ teaspoon kosher or sea salt

The first time Deanna made ricotta at home, she couldn't believe how simple it was (not to mention how incredible it tastes compared to the store-bought version). The only impediment might be not having cheesecloth on hand, but you can find it at your grocery store or any craft store or easily order it online. And in a pinch, a few coffee filters or a thin, uncolored dish towel will work just fine! The ricotta can be enjoyed as is or used in other dishes—check out the index in the back of the book for all our recipes that call for ricotta (and see this recipe's Hack on how to use up those 4 cups of leftover whey!).

Healthy Kitchen Hack:
We have lots of ways to use that whey! Mix it into waffle, pancake, or muffin batter as a substitute for the liquid. Add it to oats before cooking or mix into overnight oats. Whisk it into milk- or cream-based soups. Whirl into your favorite fruit smoothie. Most recipes that call for milk, buttermilk, or kefir will work with whey.

Set a large colander in a large bowl. Line the colander with two layers of fine cheesecloth.

In a large pot over medium heat, combine the milk and buttermilk. Stir occasionally until the curds start to separate into small white lumps from the watery liquid whey and float to the top, about 5 minutes. Continue to cook, stirring occasionally, as more curds form (the liquid will look lumpy as a thicker layer of curds continues to form on top), until the whey is opaque and thin, about an additional 5 minutes. If the whey starts to simmer, turn the heat to medium-low. Remove the pot from the heat.

Carefully strain the mixture through the cheesecloth (leave about 1 tablespoon whey in with the curds to keep the ricotta moist). Remove the colander and pour the whey into a jar or sealed container to store in the refrigerator for up to 5 days.

Scrape the ricotta curds from the cheesecloth into a bowl. Mix in the salt and either enjoy as is or season as you'd like (see our flavoring suggestions on the next page). Homemade ricotta will stay fresh in a covered container in the refrigerator for about 5 days.

Per Serving (2 tablespoons, using whole milk): **Calories: 81; Total Fat: 6g; Saturated Fat: 3g;** Cholesterol: 16mg; Sodium: 50mg; Total Carbohydrates: 1g; Fiber: 0g; Protein: 6g
Per Serving (2 tablespoons, using 2% milk): **Calories: 53; Total Fat: 3g; Saturated Fat: 2g;** Cholesterol: 16mg; Sodium: 51mg; Total Carbohydrates: 1g; Fiber: 0g; Protein: 6g

Flavor Options

Take your luscious homemade ricotta to the next level with these ingredient additions:

Classic Mediterranean Ricotta: Whisk in 1 teaspoon extra-virgin olive oil and ½ teaspoon za'atar.

Everything Ricotta: Mix in ½ teaspoon everything bagel seasoning.

Lemon Pepper Ricotta: Mix in 1 teaspoon grated lemon zest, ⅛ teaspoon black pepper, and 1 tablespoon chopped fresh chives.

Cannoli Ricotta: Go sweet with ¼ teaspoon ground cinnamon, ¼ teaspoon ground nutmeg, ½ teaspoon sugar, and ¼ teaspoon vanilla extract.

Fruit and Mint Ricotta: Mix in ¼ cup fresh or thawed frozen blueberries, ½ teaspoon honey, and 2 fresh mint leaves and stems, torn.

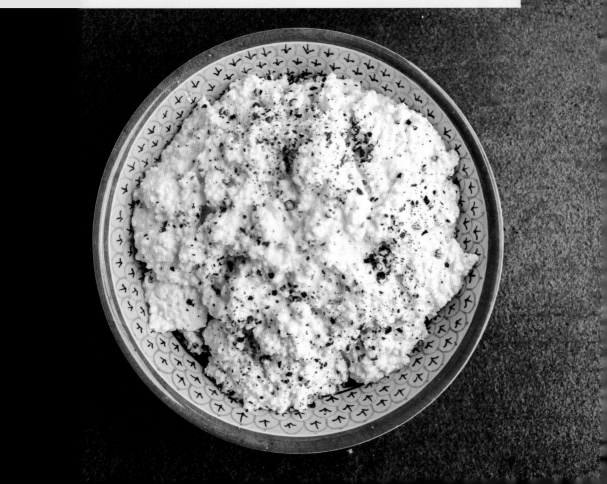

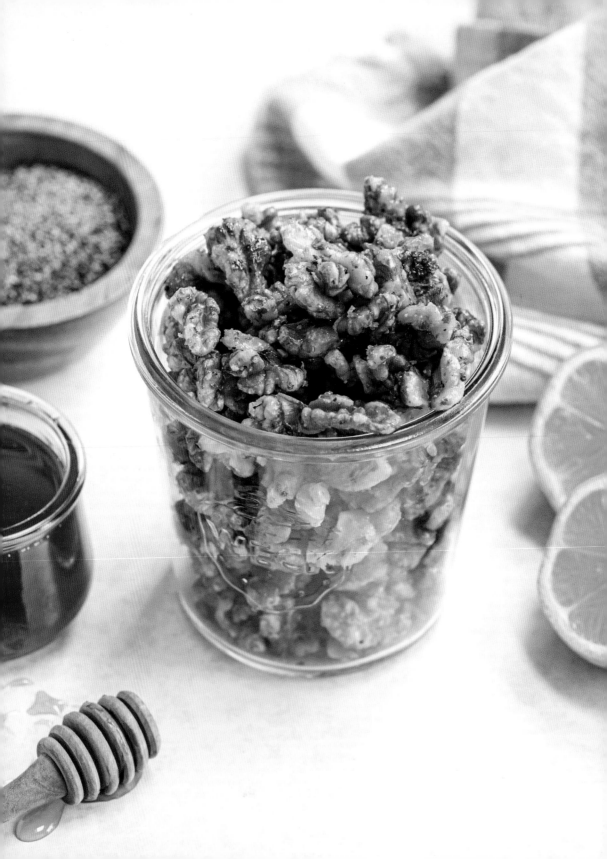

Lemon, Black Pepper, and Honey Toasted Walnuts

SERVES 6
Prep time: 5 minutes
Cook time: 10 minutes

1½ cups walnuts (whole or pieces)

¼ teaspoon kosher or sea salt

¼ teaspoon black pepper

1 lemon

1 tablespoon honey

This snack is so quick you'll have it whipped up in time to satiate all your sweet, salty, crunchy cravings! Toss the cooled walnuts over oatmeal, mix them into salads, or serve them to guests as an appetizer and watch them disappear.

Lay a piece of parchment paper on a rimmed baking sheet or heatproof surface.

In a large skillet on the stove (heat not turned on yet), combine the walnuts, salt, and pepper. Using a Microplane or citrus zester, grate the zest from the lemon into the skillet (save the remaining lemon for another use). Turn the heat to medium. Stir frequently for about 2 minutes, until the nuts are warm (you will need an extra 1 to 2 minutes if the walnuts are coming directly out of the freezer.)

Add the honey and cook, stirring frequently, until the nuts are completely coated and start to smell toasted, 2 to 3 minutes. Remove from the heat and spread the nuts on the parchment paper. Cool completely, at least 15 minutes (the nuts will still be somewhat sticky). Store in an airtight container at room temperature for about a week or freeze for about 3 months.

Healthy Kitchen Hack: Keep all your nuts fresh for longer by storing them in the freezer—it prevents them from going rancid. When you're ready to use them in a recipe, there's no need to thaw, just throw them in right from the freezer. For this recipe, use whichever nuts you have on hand or any that you may need to use up, like peanuts, pecans, pistachios, or a combination. Switch up the flavors by adding ¼ teaspoon of a Mediterranean spice such as ground cumin, ground turmeric, za'atar, smoked paprika, or ground allspice.

Per Serving: Calories: 174; Total Fat: 16g; Saturated Fat: 2g; Cholesterol: 0mg; Sodium: 81mg; Total Carbohydrates: 6g; Fiber: 2g; Protein: 4g

Antipasto Pickles

SERVES 10

Prep time: 10 minutes
plus 2 hours
refrigeration

Cook time: 10 minutes

**6 cups cut vegetables
of choice (see
headnote)**

2 garlic cloves

**3 cups white wine
vinegar or apple cider
vinegar**

¼ cup sugar

**3 tablespoons kosher
or sea salt**

**1 tablespoon dried
oregano**

**1 teaspoon fennel
seeds (optional)**

**½ teaspoon crushed
red pepper**

**¼ teaspoon black
pepper**

Antipasto is the Italian appetizer platter typically featuring cheeses, cured meats, anchovies, olives, and garlicky pickled vegetables. Here we use a quick pickling process for those veggies, which is a delectable and sustainable way to use up limp cauliflower florets, carrot sticks or coins, cucumber spears or slices, bell pepper rings or slices, green beans, cherry tomatoes, and red onion rings. In fact, wilted vegetables are actually best for pickling because they better absorb the tangy brine to deliver the most vibrant flavor. While these pickles are yummy on their own, you'll see them pop up as a flavorful ingredient throughout the book, as in our Spicy Fish Shawarma Bowls (page 225) and Toasted Squash Seeds and Cheese Board (page 61).

Divide the vegetable pieces into two quart-size mason jars or put them all in a large, heatproof glass bowl. Using the flat side of a chef's knife, press down on each garlic clove to smash, then remove the skin. Add one clove to each jar, or put both in the bowl.

In a medium saucepan over medium-high heat, combine 3 cups water, the vinegar, sugar, salt, oregano (crushed between your fingers), fennel (if using), crushed red pepper, and black pepper; stir together. Heat until the liquid boils, stirring occasionally. Carefully pour the hot brine over the vegetables. Cover the mason jars with lids or the bowl with a plate. Refrigerate the pickles for at least 2 hours. Eat within 2 weeks.

Healthy Kitchen Hack: If you purchase jarred pickles (we still buy them, too, along with making homemade), save that pickle brine to make instant cucumber pickles. Brine from dill pickles, bread and butter pickles, sweet pickles, and especially spicy pickles makes delicious, fresh cucumber pickles. Simply slice cucumbers into spears or coins, drop them in the jar with the brine, and chill overnight for the best flavor.

Per Serving: Calories: 30; Total Fat: 0g; Saturated Fat: 0g; Cholesterol: 0mg; Sodium: 270mg; Total Carbohydrates: 7g; Fiber: 1g; Protein: 1g

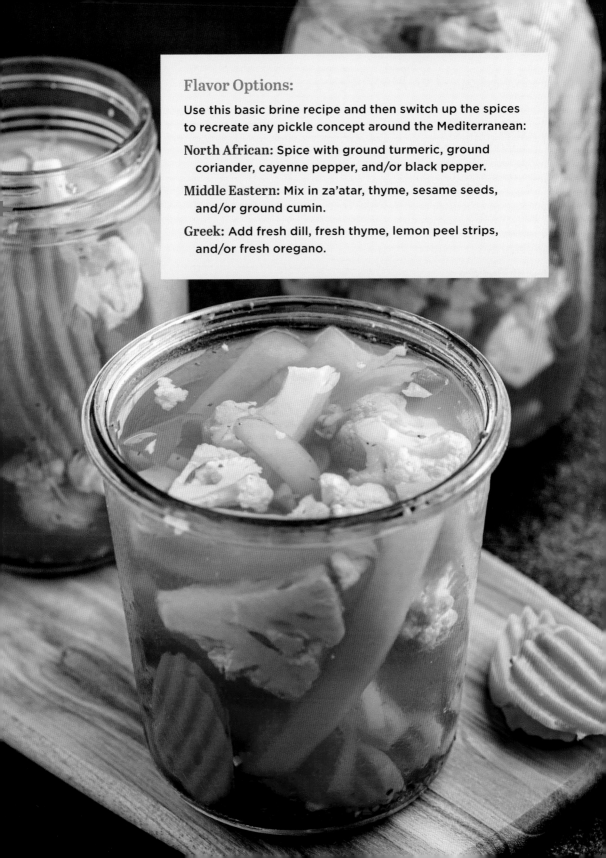

Flavor Options:

Use this basic brine recipe and then switch up the spices to recreate any pickle concept around the Mediterranean:

North African: Spice with ground turmeric, ground coriander, cayenne pepper, and/or black pepper.

Middle Eastern: Mix in za'atar, thyme, sesame seeds, and/or ground cumin.

Greek: Add fresh dill, fresh thyme, lemon peel strips, and/or fresh oregano.

Cassoulet Bean Dip

**MAKES ABOUT
2⅔ CUPS (SERVES 8)**
Prep time: 10 minutes
Cook time: 15 minutes

3 garlic cloves

4 tablespoons extra-virgin olive oil, divided

2 carrots, finely chopped

1 medium onion (any type), finely chopped

2 thyme sprigs
or ½ teaspoon dried thyme

2 (15-ounce) cans cannellini or great northern beans, drained and liquid reserved

1 tablespoon tomato paste

½ teaspoon smoked paprika

½ teaspoon black pepper

1½ tablespoons red wine vinegar

¼ cup panko bread crumbs

Out of necessity, cooks from past centuries were the ultimate sustainable chefs, using up every scrap of the food they worked hard to buy or to produce themselves. Case in point: in the South of France, residents made cassoulet. The dish is named after the vessel in which it bakes, a deep, round earthenware pot with slanting sides. Traditionally, cassoulet is made from white beans and vegetables, flavored with bits of sausage and herbs, then thickened by reducing the starchy bean cooking water. For our dip version, you can start with dried beans that simmer for an hour as the French do (see our Hack), or make our 15-minute version using canned beans that come with the bonus starchy bean liquid. To keep it vegan (and you won't believe it is!), we use smoked paprika instead of meat, but if desired, you can serve leftover cooked or cured sausage alongside the dip with raw vegetables, crusty bread, pita bread, and/or whole-grain crackers.

Using the flat side of a chef's knife, press down on each garlic clove to smash, then remove the skin.

In a small saucepan over medium-low heat, heat 1 tablespoon oil. Add the smashed garlic cloves and cook, stirring frequently to prevent burning, for 1 minute. Turn off the heat, but leave the pan on the stove for the garlic to steep in the oil while preparing the rest of the dish.

In a Dutch oven or large stockpot over medium heat, heat 2 tablespoons oil. Add the carrots, onion, and the leaves from the fresh thyme (or dried thyme, if using); cook, stirring occasionally, for 8 minutes or until the onions are translucent. Reduce the heat to medium-low, add 2 tablespoons of the reserved bean liquid, and stir. Cover and cook until the carrots are just fork-tender, 5 to 6 minutes.

While the vegetables cook, remove the garlic from the oil (keeping the pan with the oil on the stove). Mince the garlic.

Move the vegetables to the outer edges of the Dutch oven. Pour in the remaining 1 tablespoon oil and swirl it around. Add the minced garlic, tomato paste, smoked paprika, and pepper; cook until fragrant, 3 to 4 minutes.

Add the beans, ½ cup of the reserved bean liquid, and the vinegar; cook, stirring occasionally, until warmed through, 2 to 3 minutes. Remove from the heat.

For a smooth dip, add an additional 2 to 3 tablespoons of reserved bean liquid and, using an immersion blender, puree all the ingredients in the pot (or add the contents of the pot and the extra bean liquid to a food processor, process, and then return to the pot). If you want to keep the dip chunky, skip the pureeing step and simply mash some of the beans in the pan with the back of your mixing spoon.

Turn the burner under the garlic oil skillet to medium heat. Add the bread crumbs and cook, stirring frequently, until golden and toasted, 2½ to 3 minutes. Remove from the heat and scrape the toasted bread crumbs over the warm or room-temperature dip in the pot. Transfer to a serving dish and serve.

Healthy Kitchen Hack: Make this dip from a super budget-friendly bag of dried beans! Soak 1 pound dried cannellini or great northern beans overnight according to the package directions. Drain and set aside. Follow the recipe instructions above up to and including cooking the onions, carrots, and thyme in a Dutch oven. Then, add 6 cups water and the soaked beans and bring to a boil. Reduce the heat to maintain a simmer; partially cover, and cook, stirring occasionally, until the beans are tender, 1½ to 2 hours. Add 1 teaspoon salt. Continue with the instructions above to cook the minced garlic, tomato paste, smoked paprika, and pepper in oil (doubling these ingredients since this method makes about 6 cups). Add red wine vinegar to taste. If desired, toast the panko in garlic oil as above. You could also serve this as a side of beans or a main dish.

Per Serving (about ⅓ cup dip): **Calories: 172; Total Fat: 7g; Saturated Fat: 1g; Cholesterol: 0mg; Sodium: 252mg; Total Carbohydrates: 22g; Fiber: 5g; Protein: 6g**

"My husband said we should add this to our weekly dinner rotation, he liked it that much! Even my kids said they'd eat it as their main dish with a loaf of their favorite bread and a salad."

—Ava from Palm Beach, FL

Swirled Beet and Lemon Yogurt Dip

**MAKES ABOUT
2 CUPS (SERVES 8)**
Prep time: 10 minutes

1½ cups canned or jarred sliced beets (plain or pickled)

1 lemon

2 tablespoons chopped fresh dill fronds and stems, divided

3 teaspoons extra-virgin olive oil, divided

2 teaspoons honey, divided

¼ teaspoon kosher or sea salt, divided

¼ teaspoon black pepper, divided

1 cup plain 2% Greek yogurt

Cut-up raw vegetables and toasted pita bread or bagels, cut into bite-size pieces, for serving

Deanna was never a fan of beets until adulthood when she had fresh beets that were slow roasted and perfectly seasoned. Still, it took her a few more years to acquire an appreciation for the taste and convenience of canned and jarred cooked beets—and now, this vibrant dip is one of her favorite ways to feature them. Canned beets are time savers, energy savers (no need to turn on that oven for an hour!), and also a great swap when fresh beets are out of season. Avoid food waste and serve this dip with any bread you have on its last days of freshness—simply toast it for an extra layer of flavor and texture.

Drain the beets (if using pickled beets, save the pickling juice—see the Hack), then transfer to a blender. Using a Microplane or citrus zester, grate the zest from the lemon into the blender, then cut the lemon in half and squeeze in 1 tablespoon of juice. (Save the remaining juice for another use.) Add 1 tablespoon chopped dill, 2 teaspoons oil, 1 teaspoon honey, ⅛ teaspoon salt, and ⅛ teaspoon pepper. Puree until smooth.

Spoon the yogurt into one side of a small bowl. Carefully pour the beet puree into the other side. With a butter knife, slowly swirl the yogurt into the beet puree, moving across and back, until it's mixed to your liking (you can do a few swirls or mix until the yogurt is completely incorporated into the beet puree). Drizzle with the remaining 1 teaspoon each oil and honey, then swirl. Top with the remaining 1 tablespoon chopped dill and remaining ⅛ teaspoon each salt and pepper. Serve with your favorite dippers.

Healthy Kitchen Hack: Pickled canned or jarred beets are packaged in a brine that typically includes sugar, vinegar, and a variety of spices. Think of that liquid as ruby-red gold—it's a flavor bomb that can be whisked with olive oil to make an instant salad dressing, mixed into potato or pasta salads, or stirred into our Made-in-Minutes Homemade Ricotta (page 48) to make a tangy sandwich spread.

Per Serving (about ¼ cup dip alone): Calories: 51, Total Fat: 2g; Saturated Fat: 1g; Cholesterol: 3mg; Sodium: 127mg; Total Carbohydrates: 5g; Fiber: 1g; Protein: 3g

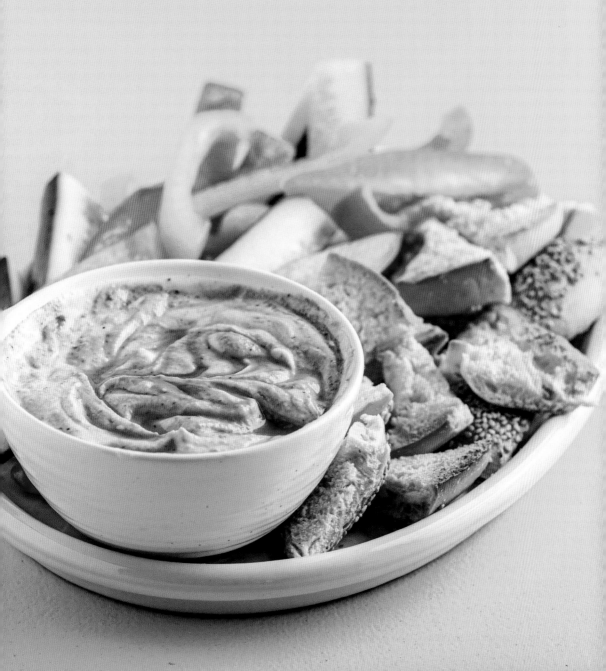

Silky-Smooth Black Pepper and Za'atar Eggplant Dip

MAKES APPROXIMATELY 2 CUPS (SERVES 6)
Prep time: 10 minutes
Cook time: 15 minutes

1 (1-pound) globe eggplant

1 lemon

2 tablespoons plus 1 teaspoon extra-virgin olive oil, divided

1½ teaspoons za'atar

½ teaspoon kosher or sea salt

½ teaspoon black pepper, plus more for serving

¼ teaspoon garlic powder

¼ teaspoon crushed red pepper

1 (15-ounce) can cannellini beans, drained and liquid reserved

4 tablespoons thinly sliced scallions (green onions), green and white parts, divided
Save the roots! See page 70

4 tablespoons chopped fresh cilantro or other herb, leaves and stems, divided

1 tablespoon tahini or peanut butter

Fresh cut vegetables, torn lavash bread, and/or Antipasto Pickles (page 52), for dipping

To celebrate finishing the manuscript of their second Mediterranean diet cookbook, Deanna and Serena met up in Philadelphia and splurged on dinner at Zahav, a lauded Israeli restaurant. One of the many dishes they swooned over was a luxurious creamy eggplant spread (a version of baba ghanoush)—they were tempted to lick the bowl! Inspired by that memorable meal, Serena created the spread with a tantalizing combination of za'atar seasoning, scallions, and cilantro. When eggplant is broiled and then pureed, it's transformed—it takes on a silky texture and creamy taste, which are a lovely contrast to the sharp black pepper and the tart lemon.

Arrange the top oven rack about 4 inches under the broiler. Preheat the broiler to high. Coat a large rimmed baking sheet with cooking spray.

Cut the stem off the eggplant. Cut the eggplant lengthwise into 4 to 6 long slabs (about ½ inch thick), but do not peel. Set aside.

Using a Microplane or citrus zester, grate the zest from the lemon into a medium bowl; cut the lemon in half and squeeze in the juice. Whisk in 2 tablespoons oil, the za'atar, salt, black pepper, garlic powder, and crushed red pepper. Brush both sides of the eggplant slabs with the lemon dressing, then set aside the remaining dressing.

Arrange the eggplant slabs on the prepared baking sheet. (If any end pieces are mainly eggplant skin with little flesh, dress and broil those too, but watch them— they'll cook faster, so be careful not to burn.) Broil for 5 minutes, then flip the slabs with tongs and broil until the eggplant flesh softens and begins to get brown in spots, an additional 5 to 7 minutes. Remove from the oven and cool on a wire rack for about 5 minutes.

Roughly chop the eggplant and then toss into a food processor or high-powered blender. Add the reserved lemon dressing, beans, 3 tablespoons scallions, 3 tablespoons cilantro, and the tahini. Process until smooth and, if needed, add 1 to 2 tablespoons of the reserved bean liquid to achieve the desired consistency.

To serve, transfer the eggplant dip to a serving bowl and drizzle with the remaining 1 teaspoon olive oil. Top with the remaining 1 tablespoon each scallions and cilantro and several grinds of black pepper. Serve with your favorite dippers.

Note: Peanut butter may be substituted for tahini, but the recipe will no longer be nut-free.

Healthy Kitchen Hack: Here are more ways to enjoy this dip: Spread it on sandwiches or serve it alongside our Zucchini, Carrot, and Gorgonzola Patties (page 173). Turn it into a soup by adding water or our Veggie Scraps Broth (page 120), then serve it the Middle Eastern way—as a cold soup with a dollop of yogurt.

Per Serving (about ⅓ cup dip alone): Calories: 146; Total Fat: 9g; Saturated Fat: 1g; Cholesterol: 0mg; Sodium: 175mg; Total Carbohydrates: 15g; Fiber: 4g; Protein: 4g

"This dip was a big hit! We loved how silky-smooth it was and enjoyed how the eggplant flavor came through. Even my eggplant-skeptic husband enjoyed it!"

—Jessica from Silver Spring, MD

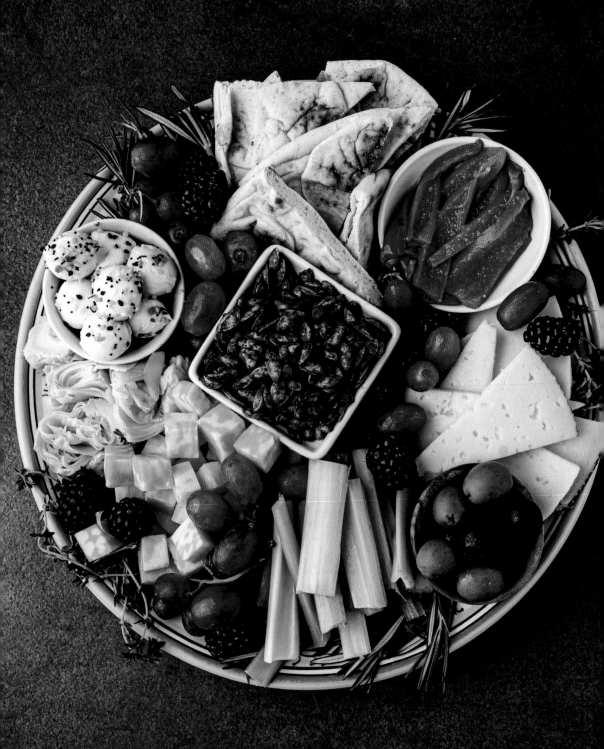

EGG-FREE, NUT-FREE, VEGETARIAN

Toasted Squash Seeds and Cheese Board

SERVES 8
Prep time: 20 minutes
Cook time: 15 minutes

Save the seeds! While it's fairly common practice to scoop and toast pumpkin seeds when we're carving jack-o'-lanterns for Halloween, other squash seeds don't often get the same type of love. So, the next time you cook a whole butternut, acorn, spaghetti, Hubbard, or delicata squash, reserve the seeds for this enticing appetizer (or full meal if you choose). Of course, you can enjoy these sweet and spicy seeds on their as own as a snack, but we like to serve them instead of (or alongside) nuts in a traditional Mediterranean cheese board spread—another great way to use up the cheeses, meats, veggies, and/or fruit that are hanging out in your fridge. Psst! Need a squash recipe so you have leftover seeds? Try our Rosemary and Chive Whipped Butternut Squash with Mascarpone Swirl (page 89).

½ cup squash seeds of choice (see headnote)

2 teaspoons extra-virgin olive oil

2 teaspoons honey

½ teaspoon ground cinnamon

½ teaspoon smoked paprika

¼ teaspoon kosher or sea salt

¼ teaspoon black pepper

FOR THE CHEESE BOARD

40 small pita breads, baguette slices, multigrain bread, and/or crackers

4 cups cut raw seasonal vegetables (broccoli, cauliflower, mushrooms, carrots, celery, cucumbers, bell peppers, etc.)

4 cups seasonal fruit (sliced peaches, plums, nectarines, apples, pears, grapes, berries, cherries, etc.)

2 cups cut/cubed cheese (feta, fresh mozzarella, Manchego, Asiago, Gorgonzola, goat cheese, etc.)

1 cup dried fruit (figs, apricots, raisins, prunes, cherries, etc.)

2 cups jarred or canned vegetables (olives, quartered artichokes, roasted red peppers, mushrooms, Antipasto Pickles (page 52), etc.)

Herb sprigs, for garnish (optional)

Optional additions: Pumpkin Hummus (page 63), Swirled Beet and Lemon Yogurt Dip (page 56), or Silky-Smooth Black Pepper and Za'atar Eggplant Dip (page 58)

To make the toasted squash seeds, preheat the oven to 375°F. Coat a large rimmed baking sheet with cooking spray or line it with parchment paper.

In a medium bowl, using your hands, mix the squash seeds, oil, honey, cinnamon, smoked paprika, salt, and pepper until the seeds are completely coated.

continued

Spread the seeds evenly on the prepared baking sheet. Bake for 10 minutes and check the seeds; if they are not yet completely golden brown, continue to bake for an additional 2 to 5 minutes (keep a close eye on the seeds as they burn easily). Keep in mind that squash seeds vary in size—for example, butternut seeds are smaller than pumpkin. Smaller seeds will toast up (and burn!) faster, while pumpkin seeds may take 5 to 15 minutes longer depending on your oven and your "toastiness" preference. Cool for 10 minutes.

While the seeds toast and then cool, arrange your cheese board. (Here's an idea: Instead of a wooden board, Deanna usually covers one of her large rimmed baking sheets with parchment paper for ease of serving and cleanup. Choose whichever setup you like!) Set an empty vessel (like a small glass bowl, ramekin, or a shallow teacup) in the center for your seeds when they've cooled. Arrange all the bread, vegetables, fruit, cheese, and dried fruit in piles on the platter. Put "wetter" ingredients like fresh mozzarella, olives, jarred roasted red peppers, or optional dips in small containers on your platter. If you have fresh herbs on hand, scatter a few sprigs around for color. Serve with small plates and mini spoons and forks, if you have them.

Healthy Kitchen Hack: Ensure that your squash seeds turn out sensational, spiced, and toasted with these tips. You can skip washing off the squash "guts" and patting them dry since the pulpy flesh adds extra flavor. And once in the oven, there's no need to stir them, but you do need to watch them. After 10 minutes, check on them through the oven door window every minute until they are golden brown—the cooking time will depend on the size of the seeds and how toasty you like them.

Per Serving (1 tablespoon toasted seeds only): Calories: 61; Total Fat: 7g; Saturated Fat: 1g; Cholesterol: 0mg; Sodium: 61mg; Total Carbohydrates: 3g; Fiber: 1g; Protein: 3g

Per Serving (1 tablespoon toasted seeds with ⅛ of each of the cheese board components): Calories: 319; Total Fat: 16g; Saturated Fat: 6g; Cholesterol: 22mg; Sodium: 575mg; Total Carbohydrates: 34g; Fiber: 7g; Protein: 14g

Pumpkin Hummus

**MAKES ABOUT
2¼ CUPS (SERVES 6)**
Prep time: 10 minutes

½ (15-ounce) can
pumpkin puree

1 (15-ounce) can
chickpeas, drained
and liquid reserved

1 lemon

2 tablespoons extra-
virgin olive oil

2 tablespoons tahini
or creamy peanut
butter

¼ teaspoon kosher or
sea salt

Winter squashes like pumpkin, butternut, acorn, and spaghetti squash are seasonal favorites in Mediterranean regions as they thrive in sandy soil and warm climates. While we've been known to cook whole pumpkins when in season—check out Serena's Whole Pumpkin Cheesy Gratin (page 181)—you can't beat the convenience and shelf-life of canned pumpkin (make sure to buy pure 100% pumpkin, not pumpkin pie filling, which includes sugar and other flavorings). Mix it into our super easy hummus recipe for a boost of nutrition, color, and flavor. Enjoy with traditional hummus accompaniments or serve on our Toasted Squash Seeds and Cheese Board (page 61).

Scoop the canned pumpkin into a blender or food processor. Add ¼ cup of the reserved chickpea liquid and process until smooth.

Using a Microplane or citrus zester, grate the zest from the lemon into the blender; cut the lemon in half and squeeze in 1 tablespoon of lemon juice. (Use the remaining lemon juice, pumpkin, and chickpea liquid to make a double batch of hummus or save them for another use.) Add the drained chickpeas, oil, tahini, and salt to the blender and process until smooth. For an even lighter, fluffier texture, add another 1 to 2 tablespoons chickpea liquid to achieve your preferred consistency.

Note: Peanut butter may be substituted for tahini, but the recipe will no longer be nut-free.

Healthy Kitchen Hack: Flavor up your pumpkin hummus! For a sweeter taste, blend in 1 teaspoon ground cinnamon and use as a morning toast topping or a mix-in for hot cereal. Or go the savory route and blend in 1 tablespoon za'atar; serve with warm pita and raw veggies or use as a yummy sandwich spread.

"This hummus was fun to make and really delicious. My husband loved it too, and even started using it as a dip for his roasted almonds!"

—**Liz from Collegeville, PA**

Per Serving (6 tablespoons): Calories: 145; Total Fat: 8g; Saturated Fat: 1g; Cholesterol: 0mg; Sodium: 305mg; Total Carbohydrates: 14g; Fiber: 4g; Protein: 5g

Loaded Greek Potato Chips

SERVES 4
Prep time: 10 minutes
Cook time: 20 minutes

2 (8-ounce) russet
potatoes, well
scrubbed

2 tablespoons extra-
virgin olive oil

1 teaspoon dried
oregano

½ teaspoon kosher or
sea salt

¼ teaspoon black
pepper

1 cucumber, unpeeled,
cut in half

⅔ cup plain 2% Greek
yogurt

4 tablespoons
chopped fresh dill or
other herb, leaves and
stems, divided

1 garlic clove, minced

¼ cup diced red onion

4 ounces feta cheese,
crumbled

These irresistibly crispy potato chips are fun to make—
often—especially when you discover how easy they are. Keep
them simple with just olive oil, salt, and pepper, or turn them
into this appetizer with tons of toppings, including homemade
tzatziki. The combo of fresh dill, sharp onions, and tangy
feta along with textures of super crunchy potatoes, crisp
cukes, and smooth creamy yogurt going on in your mouth is
as much fun as the Tsamiko dance Serena once learned at a
Greek wedding!

Arrange the oven racks to the upper-middle and lower-
middle positions. Preheat the oven to 400°F. Coat two
large rimmed baking sheets with cooking spray.

Slice the potatoes into thin chips using a mandoline
(carefully!), a knife, or a spiralizer with the flat blade
(making "ribbon" chips about 3 inches long). In a large
bowl, toss the potato chips with the oil, oregano, salt,
and pepper until well coated. Spread the chips evenly
between the prepared baking sheets and arrange so that
the potatoes are barely overlapping.

Put both sheets in the oven and bake for 10 minutes.
Remove from the oven and, using tongs, flip the chips,
then return the sheets to the opposite racks. Bake for an
additional 10 to 12 minutes or until the chips are crispy.

While the chips cook, shred half of the cucumber
with a box grater or finely chop with a knife. In a small
bowl, stir together the shredded cucumber, yogurt,
3 tablespoons dill, and garlic to make a tzatziki sauce.
Dice the remaining half of the cucumber and set aside.

Transfer the cooked chips from one sheet onto the
other sheet for serving (or transfer all the chips to a
serving platter). Spoon the tzatziki sauce over the chips,
then sprinkle with the diced cucumber and onion. Top
with the crumbled feta and remaining 1 tablespoon dill
and serve immediately.

Healthy Kitchen Hack: For years, Serena resisted the
food bloggers (and Deanna!), who told her she needed
a spiralizer. But then she picked one up at a garage sale
(an eco-friendly way to obtain a new kitchen tool) and

discovered it was more than worth it for these chips alone. And since this nifty gadget has so many slicing options, she sometimes changes this recipe into Loaded Greek Shoestring Fries by using the fine shredding blade to spiralize the potatoes into thin strings, about 12 inches long.

Per Serving: Calories: 236; Total Fat: 14g; Saturated Fat: 6g; Cholesterol: 28mg; Sodium: 522mg; Total Carbohydrates: 20g; Fiber: 2g; Protein: 10g

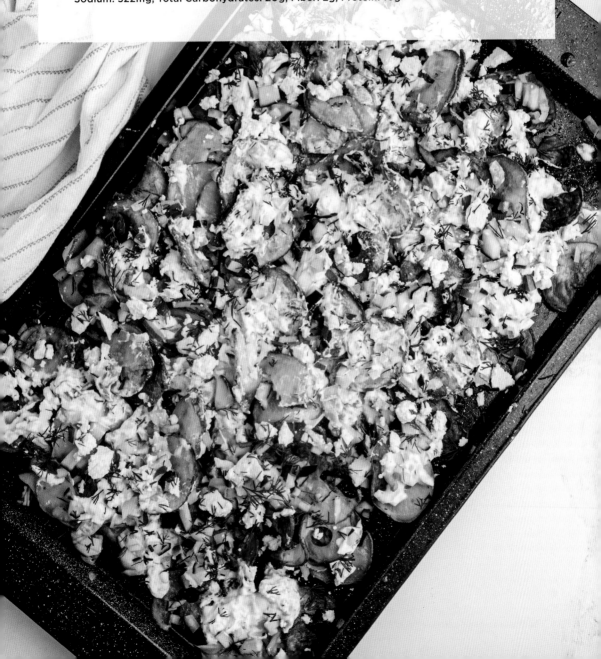

Vanilla and Fruit Seeded Granola Bars

MAKES 10 BARS (SERVES 10)
Prep time: 15 minutes
Cook time: 30 minutes

1 orange

½ cup dried fruit of choice, chopped if large

2 tablespoons ground flaxseed

⅓ cup plus 1 tablespoon tahini, divided

⅓ cup plus 1 teaspoon honey, divided

1½ teaspoons vanilla extract, divided

1 teaspoon ground cinnamon

¼ teaspoon kosher or sea salt

1 cup gluten-free quick or old-fashioned oats

1 cup mixed seeds of choice (see headnote)

Because seeds contain all the components of what will become a whole plant, they are loaded with fiber, monounsaturated fats, protein, antioxidants, and more. Seeds, especially sesame seeds, pine nuts (actually seeds!), and pumpkin seeds, are used throughout the Mediterranean region to add protein and crunch to main dishes and snacks. And, as a bonus for sustainability, they typically require much less water than tree nuts to grow. So, get out of your nut rut and use more seeds! We set out to pack as many crunchy seeds as possible into these chewy granola bars and ended up making ours with a combo of sesame, chia, sunflower, pumpkin, and squash seeds—but you can use just one or two kinds if that's what you have. The result is a vanilla- and orange-scented baked and frosted treat that tastes so yummy, you may forget it's power-packed with stellar nutrition, too.

Preheat the oven to 325°F. Coat a 9-inch square baking dish with cooking spray. Line the baking dish with a rectangular sheet of parchment paper that hangs over two opposite sides, then coat the parchment with cooking spray.

Using a Microplane or citrus zester, grate the zest from the orange into a stand mixer bowl (or regular mixing bowl). Cut the orange in half and squeeze 1 tablespoon orange juice into a separate small bowl and set aside. (Enjoy the remaining part of the orange as a snack!)

Add the dried fruit, flaxseed, and ½ cup boiling or hot water to the bowl and let sit for 5 minutes to hydrate the fruit and flaxseed. Add ⅓ cup tahini, ⅓ cup honey, 1 teaspoon vanilla, and the cinnamon and salt. Using the paddle attachment (or a wooden spoon), mix until well combined. Scrape down the sides and add the oats; mix until combined. Add the seeds; mix until just combined.

Pour the mixture into the prepared pan and spread with a cooking spray–coated silicone scraper until the mixture is evenly distributed. Bake for 25 to 30 minutes or until the top is golden brown, the edges are firm, and the center gives slightly when pressed.

While the bars bake, add the remaining 1 tablespoon tahini, remaining 1 teaspoon honey, and remaining ½ teaspoon vanilla to the bowl with the orange juice; whisk until combined. Once the bars are out of the oven, drizzle this glaze over the warm bars and spread evenly so the glaze soaks in and makes them slightly shiny. Cool completely in the pan on a wire rack.

Using the parchment paper overhang as handles, remove the bars from the pan. Cut into 10 rectangular bars and serve.

Notes: Peanut butter may be substituted for tahini, but the recipe will no longer be nut-free. The Toasted Squash Seeds from page 61 could also be used as the seeds of choice.

Healthy Kitchen Hack: Want to bake but you're out of eggs? Sub in a "flax egg" as we do with these bars. This swap adds monounsaturated fats and fiber to recipes while mimicking the thickening and moistening properties of a chicken egg. For each egg a recipe calls for, whisk together 1 tablespoon ground flaxseed with 3 tablespoons warm water. Let sit for 5 minutes to hydrate before adding to a batter. Flax eggs work well for batter recipes such as pancakes, quick breads, brownies, muffins, and cookies, but not for meringues, omelets, or egg-based dishes.

Per Serving: Calories: 240; Total Fat: 13g; Saturated Fat: 1.8g; Cholesterol: 0mg; Sodium: 54mg; Total Carbohydrates: 29g; Fiber: 3g; Protein: 7g

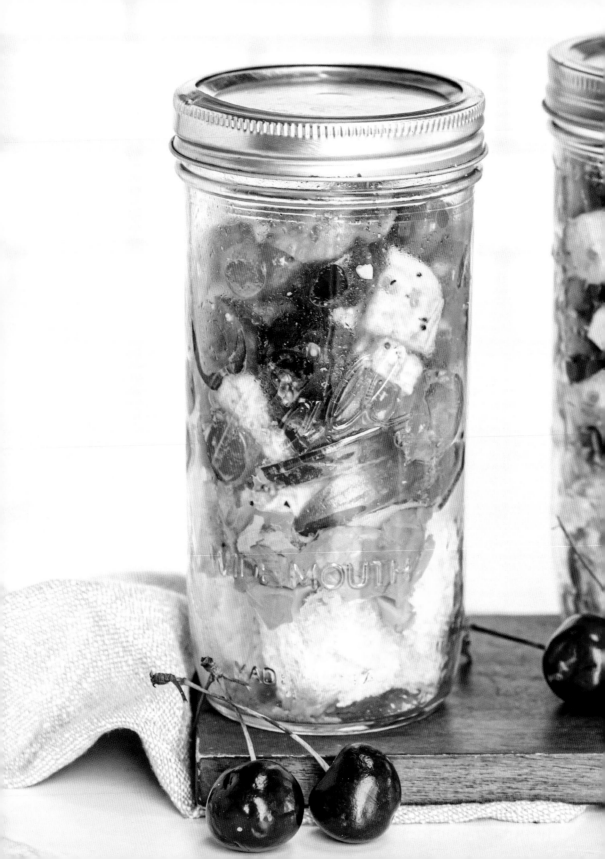

Salads

Honey, Orange, and Scallion Vinaigrette over Romaine

SERVES 6
Prep time: 10 minutes

1 (11-ounce) can mandarins in light syrup, drained and liquid reserved

4 scallions (green onions), green and white parts, thinly sliced
Save the stems! See the Hack

¼ cup extra-virgin olive oil

2 tablespoons white wine vinegar or rice wine vinegar

1 tablespoon Dijon mustard

2 teaspoons honey

¼ teaspoon kosher or sea salt

¼ teaspoon black pepper

2 heads romaine lettuce, chopped (about 10 cups)
Save the stems! See the Hack

Canned fruits, like mandarin oranges, are Mediterranean staples in our recipes because of their versatility and long shelf lives. Plus, there's so much you can do with that leftover liquid after draining. Along with oranges and this vinaigrette, Deanna likes to toss in our Lemon, Black Pepper, and Honey Toasted Walnuts (page 51) with some shaved Pecorino or Parmesan cheese. Be sure to check out this recipe's Healthy Kitchen Hack highlighting how super easy it is to grow a few of this salad's ingredients!

Pour 3 tablespoons of the reserved mandarin orange liquid into a blender (save the remainder to use in other dressings or mix with seltzer for a light citrus drink). Set the oranges aside until the salad is ready to serve.

To the blender, add the scallions, oil, vinegar, mustard, honey, salt, and pepper. Blend until smooth.

Right before serving, put the romaine in a serving bowl. Toss in the drained oranges and drizzle half of the dressing over the salad. Toss to coat.

Store the remaining dressing in a sealed container in the refrigerator for up to 7 days. Use the leftover dressing on a future salad or toss it with small shaped pasta like we do with our Israeli Couscous "Pasta Salad" on page 85.

Healthy Kitchen Hack: Did you know you can regrow scallions and romaine lettuce from their trimmed root ends? Even as a self-professed "black thumb," Deanna has had much success with this method. Cut the romaine stems about 2 inches from their ends and the scallion white roots about 1 inch from their ends. Arrange them standing up in about 1 inch of water in a small glass or dish (Deanna uses a shot glass for scallions) and set by a sunny window. Change the water almost daily, and you'll have new scallion sprouts to harvest in about a week and new romaine in 10 to 12 days!

Per Serving: Calories: 158; Total Fat: 10g; Saturated Fat: 1g; Cholesterol: 0mg; Sodium: 166mg; Total Carbohydrates: 18g; Fiber: 5g; Protein: 3g

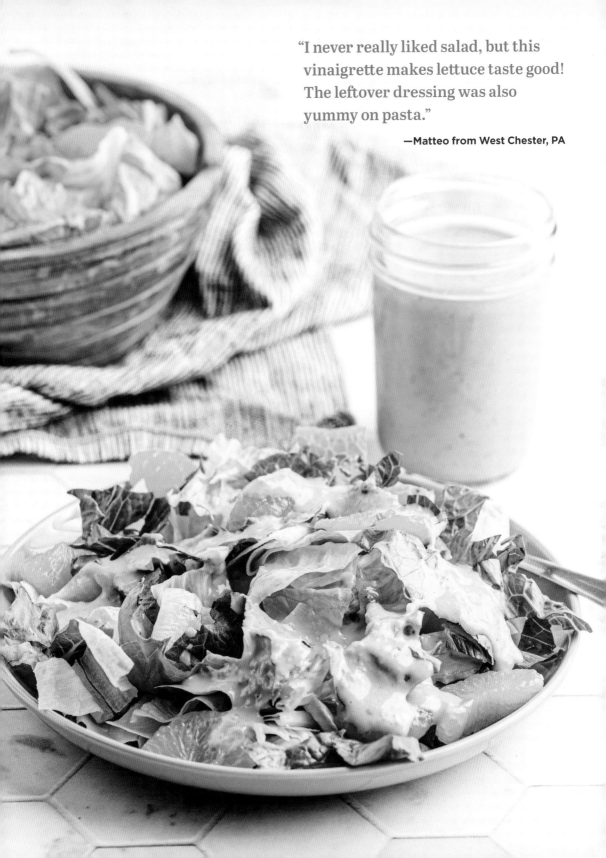

"I never really liked salad, but this vinaigrette makes lettuce taste good! The leftover dressing was also yummy on pasta."

—Matteo from West Chester, PA

Summer Cherry Caprese Panzanella Salad in Jars

SERVES 6
Prep time: 15 minutes

1 lemon

1 cup thinly sliced red onion

1 pint cherries, pitted, stemmed, and cut in half (about 1½ cups)

1½ cups chopped tomatoes or cherry/grape tomatoes, cut in half

8 ounces fresh mozzarella cheese, cubed

2 tablespoons extra-virgin olive oil

1 tablespoon balsamic vinegar

¼ teaspoon kosher or sea salt

¼ teaspoon black pepper

3 cups cubed baguette or other crusty bread (1-inch pieces)

1 cup fresh mint or basil (or a combination), leaves and stems, gently torn

During peak summer months, this portable salad is Deanna's favorite lunch to pack into glass jars, toss into a cooler bag, and take to the beach. It's quick to whip up and super versatile. You can use any combination of fresh seasonal fruit you may have on hand beyond cherries—like berries, balled melon, diced peaches, chopped plums, and/or grapes—with any crusty or multigrain bread that may be getting too hard. Deanna sometimes tosses in kernels from leftover corn on the cob, which adds even more nutrition and color to this vibrant salad.

Using a Microplane or citrus zester, grate the zest from the lemon into a medium bowl. Cut the lemon in half and squeeze the juice into the bowl. Stir in the onion and set aside for at least 5 minutes. (This step helps tame the pungency of the onion.)

In a large mixing or serving bowl, toss together the cherries, tomatoes, mozzarella, oil, vinegar, salt, and pepper. Add the onion with the lemon juice and zest, then toss again. Refrigerate until ready to transfer to large glass jars with lids. (If you're eating this at home, when ready to serve, simply add the cubed bread and mint or basil to the bowl and toss well.)

When you are ready to pack the salads, arrange the cubed bread in the bottom of two or more jars (see the Hack). Layer on the mint or basil and then the cherry tomato mixture, leaving about 2 inches air space at the top. Cover and pack in a cooler. Before eating, shake vigorously until well blended.

Healthy Kitchen Hack: While Deanna's husband often grumbles about the jars taking up space in their cupboards, both she and Serena love to repurpose empty condiment jars. From large pickle or mayonnaise jars to smaller ones from jam or mustard, they use them for portable meals like this recipe or for leftover food storage. You can also look for mason and Ball canning jars at yard sales—a super inexpensive way to recycle and repurpose!

Per Serving: Calories: 262; Total Fat: 13g; Saturated Fat: 6g; Cholesterol: 30mg; Sodium: 408mg; Total Carbohydrates: 25g; Fiber: 2g; Protein: 10g

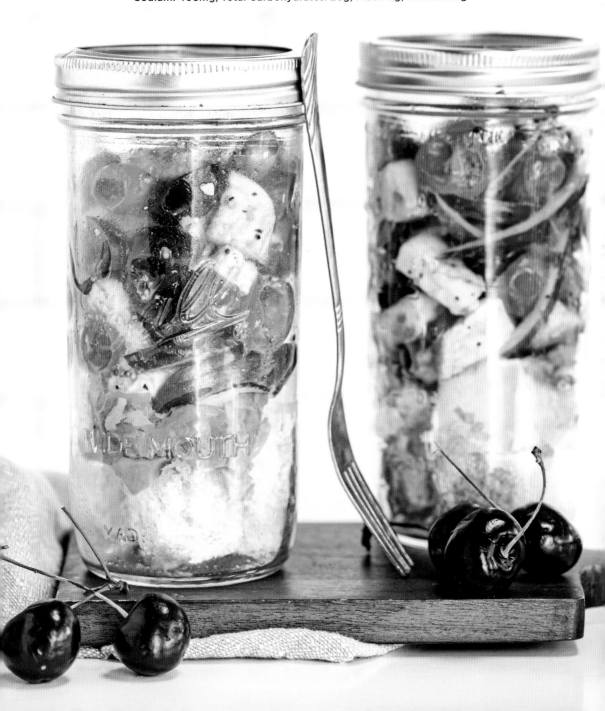

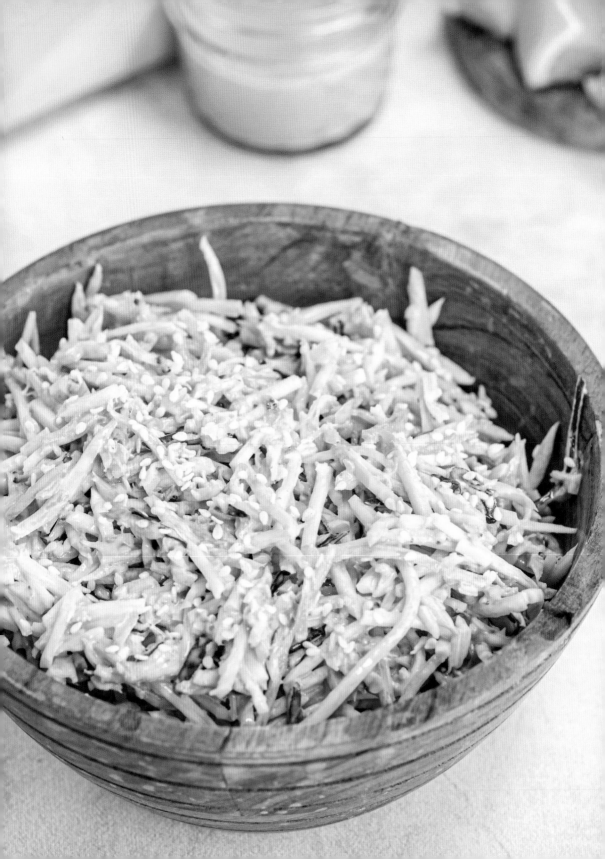

Tahini Use-Up-Those-Veggies Slaw

SERVES 6
Prep time: 15 minutes

1 lemon

2 tablespoons tahini
or peanut butter

1 tablespoon extra-
virgin olive oil

1 tablespoon honey

¼ teaspoon kosher or
sea salt

6–7 cups shredded or
julienned vegetables
(see headnote)

1 tablespoon toasted
sesame seeds
(optional)

"My family had
never tried tahini,
but we really liked
the nutty flavor,
especially paired
with the citrus. It
was a yummy way
to use up some
older lettuce I had."

—Eliza from
Edwardsville, IL

We call this one a back-pocket recipe because it's easy to commit to memory—and it will save dinner again and again, in more ways than one. First, it's a super quick side that is bound to become a go-to favorite because of the sweet-tart, nutty dressing, using the Middle Eastern staple tahini. Second, almost any vegetable in your fridge will benefit from a drizzle of this dressing, so it's a great way to use them up. We think this slaw works particularly well with red or green cabbage, broccoli stems, zucchini, carrots, and even the white part of watermelon rinds (see the Hack)—or a combination of all of them!

Using a Microplane or citrus zester, grate the zest from the lemon into a medium bowl. Cut the lemon in half and squeeze the juice into the bowl. Whisk in the tahini, oil, honey, and salt. (If using peanut butter, you may need to add 1 tablespoon hot water to emulsify everything.) Add the shredded vegetables and toss until well coated. Sprinkle with the toasted sesame seeds, if desired. Serve immediately. If making ahead, store the dressing separately from the vegetables.

Note: Peanut butter may be substituted for tahini, but the recipe will no longer be nut-free.

Healthy Kitchen Hack: Yes, you can eat watermelon rinds! They're crunchy, refreshing, and much like the vegetable jicama in texture and flavor. Slice off the pink-red flesh (and enjoy!), then trim off the thin green part of the rind (and compost). The remaining white part is totally edible; slice or cut into matchstick pieces and use as the perfect addition to this slaw, as well as stir-fries, pasta salads, our Antipasto Pickles (page 52), and Cheesy Crab Panini (page 141).

Per Serving: Calories: 92; Total Fat: 5g; Saturated Fat: 1g; Cholesterol: 0mg; Sodium: 105mg; Total Carbohydrates: 11g; Fiber: 2g; Protein: 2g

Windowsill Herb Salad with Tomatoes and Za'atar

SERVES 6
Prep time: 15 minutes

1 lemon

1 cup thinly sliced red onion

1 garlic clove, minced

3 medium tomatoes, sliced, *or* 3 cups halved cherry tomatoes

1 teaspoon za'atar, divided

½ teaspoon kosher or sea salt, divided

½ teaspoon black pepper, divided

3 cups finely chopped fresh herbs of choice (see headnote), leaves and stems

3 cups salad greens of choice (see headnote)

2 tablespoons extra-virgin olive oil

2 teaspoons red wine vinegar

If you're like Serena, you look forward to growing a variety of vegetables and herbs in your garden every year. If you're like Deanna, you may have trouble keeping a common house plant alive. But whether you have a green or black thumb, we're confident you can have success with growing a few herbs at home by a sunny window with the Healthy Kitchen Hack following this recipe. This simple yet vibrant salad recipe features equal parts herbs (like parsley, cilantro, basil, mint, dill, and chives) and salad greens (like romaine, arugula, butter lettuce, and Bibb)—Mediterranean cuisine routinely features full cups instead of teaspoons of fresh herbs. It's also versatile enough to accommodate whatever you can "harvest" from your sill all year round, though we especially like it in the summer when tomatoes from the garden (or market) are at their very best.

Using a Microplane or citrus zester, grate the zest from the lemon into a small bowl. Cut the lemon in half and squeeze in the juice. Stir in the onion and garlic and let sit while you prepare the remaining ingredients.

In a medium bowl, toss the tomatoes with ½ teaspoon za'atar, ¼ teaspoon salt, and ¼ teaspoon pepper and set aside.

In a large serving bowl, gently toss together the fresh herbs, salad greens, onion with the lemon juice and zest, and tomatoes. In the same bowl that held the onion, whisk together the oil, vinegar, remaining ½ teaspoon za'atar, and remaining ¼ teaspoon each salt and pepper. Pour over the salad and gently toss again before serving.

Healthy Kitchen Hack: The easiest herbs to grow and maintain indoors tend to be basil, chives, mint, oregano, parsley, and rosemary. You'll have the most success at a windowsill that gets around 6 hours of sunlight a day. Read up on the best size pot if you're growing from seeds or if using seedlings. Keep the soil damp, but water the herbs sparingly. Also, be sure to try our Hack on page 70 for tips on regrowing scallions and romaine lettuce from the stems in only water—even Deanna has done this with positive results!

Per Serving: Calories: 69; Total Fat: 5g; Saturated Fat: 1g; Cholesterol: 0mg; Sodium: 174mg; Total Carbohydrates: 6g; Fiber: 2g; Protein: 1g

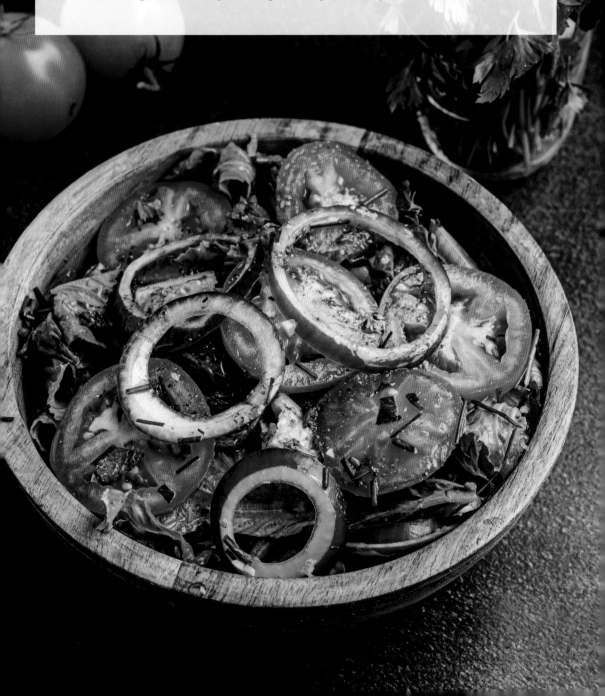

Roasted Cabbage Wedge Caesar Salad

SERVES 8
Prep time: 10 minutes
Cook time: 25 minutes

1 (2- to 2½-pound) head green or red cabbage

4 tablespoons extra-virgin olive oil, divided

½ teaspoon kosher or sea salt, divided

½ teaspoon black pepper, divided

2 slices whole-grain bread

1 small garlic clove, cut in half

1 anchovy from 1 (2-ounce) tin anchovies in olive oil
Save the extra anchovies and oil! See page 158

1 lemon

⅓ cup plain whole-milk Greek yogurt

2 teaspoons Dijon mustard

¼ cup grated Asiago or Parmesan cheeses

Roasting does something magical to cabbage. While the oven causes the veggie's natural sugars to caramelize and sweeten, roasting also creates an appealing toothsome texture that's somewhere between crunchy and soft/tender. But we could not decide whether this would be a cabbage wedge Caesar—to celebrate our new love of canned seafood—or a Mediterranean riff on the blue cheese and bacon wedge salad of trendy restaurant fame. And so, you get both options—see our gorgonzola dressing option in this recipe's Hack!

Preheat the oven to 425°F. Coat a large rimmed baking sheet with cooking spray.

Cut the cabbage head in half through the middle of the core. Cut each half into four wedges, through the core so the wedges stay intact. Arrange the eight wedges on the prepared baking sheet. Brush the wedges with 2 tablespoons oil and sprinkle with ¼ teaspoon each salt and pepper, then gently spread the leaves of the wedges slightly so air can circulate between them (but keep the leaves attached to the core). Roast for 15 to 20 minutes, until the bottoms begin to turn golden. Remove from the oven, flip the cabbage wedges, and add the pieces of bread to the baking sheet. Roast for 5 to 8 more minutes, until the cabbage is fork-tender but still firm and the bread is toasted. Cool slightly on a wire rack for 5 to 10 minutes. Rub the cut sides of the garlic halves on both sides of the toasted bread slices, then cut the bread into small croutons.

While the cabbage roasts, in a medium bowl, use a fork to mash together the garlic halves, anchovy, and remaining ¼ teaspoon each salt and pepper to form a paste. Using a Microplane or citrus zester, grate the zest from the lemon over the anchovy mixture; cut the lemon in half and squeeze in 2 tablespoons juice. (Save the remaining juice for another use.) Whisk in the yogurt and mustard, then drizzle in the remaining 2 tablespoons oil while whisking constantly.

(Alternatively, if you have a mini food processor, you could use it instead of a fork and whisk.)

Serve the cabbage wedges warm or at room temperature, topped with the dressing, croutons, and grated cheese. Or make a day ahead; chill the roasted cabbage wedges and dressing separately overnight; store the croutons in an airtight container at room temperature. Before serving, whisk the dressing to fully combine.

Healthy Kitchen Hack: Thanks to our dressing indecision, we now present you with our variation of Roasted Cabbage Wedge with Gorgonzola Cheese Dressing and Smoky Croutons. Follow the above dressing instructions with these variations: Omit the anchovy and garlic. Instead, whisk together the above amounts of lemon zest, lemon juice, ¼ teaspoon each salt and pepper, yogurt, mustard, and ⅓ cup crumbled Gorgonzola. As for the croutons, instead of rubbing the toasted bread with garlic, lightly coat both sides with cooking spray and then sprinkle both sides with ¼ teaspoon smoked paprika for a smoky "bacon" flavor. Cut into croutons.

Per Serving: **Calories: 144; Total Fat: 9g; Saturated Fat: 2g; Cholesterol: 4mg; Sodium: 285mg; Total Carbohydrates: 14g; Fiber: 3g; Protein: 5g**

Broiled Halloumi over Mint Cucumber Salad

SERVES 4
Prep time: 5 minutes
Cook time: 10 minutes

1 lemon

1 cup thinly sliced red onion

3 tablespoons whole-wheat flour, white whole-wheat flour, or all-purpose flour

½ teaspoon black pepper, divided

¼ teaspoon smoked paprika

8 ounces halloumi cheese, cut into 8 slices

¼ teaspoon kosher or sea salt

2 tablespoons extra-virgin olive oil

6 cups salad greens

1 cup fresh mint, leaves and stems, torn

1 English cucumber, unpeeled, sliced

Originating from the island of Cyprus, halloumi cheese is like a lovely combination of creamy mozzarella and salty feta. Also known as "grilling cheese," halloumi melts at a higher temperature than other cheeses, so it's ideal for broiling into toasty golden slabs of slightly firm and melty goodness. In this recipe, we feature it over a bright, lemony mint salad, but feel free to eat a piece hot right out of the oven (we usually can't resist)!

Arrange the top oven rack about 4 inches under the broiler. Preheat the broiler to high. Coat a large rimmed baking sheet with cooking spray.

Using a Microplane or citrus zester, grate the zest from the lemon into a large bowl. Cut the lemon in half and squeeze in 2 tablespoons lemon juice. (Save the remaining juice for another use.) Stir in the onion and set aside. (This step helps tame the pungency of the onion.)

In a shallow bowl, whisk together the flour, ¼ teaspoon pepper, and smoked paprika. Press a slice of cheese into the flour mixture on both sides and shake off any excess. Transfer to the prepared baking sheet. Repeat with the remaining halloumi slices, arranging them down the center of the baking sheet so they will be directly under the heat source. Lightly coat the tops with cooking spray. Broil for 3 to 4 minutes, until golden (keep an eye on them to prevent burning). Flip each piece, then broil 2 to 4 more minutes, until golden on the other side.

While the halloumi cooks, add the salt and remaining ¼ teaspoon pepper to the bowl with the onion. Whisk in the oil. Add the salad greens, mint, and cucumber. Toss and coat with the dressing. Divide the salad among four plates and top each with two broiled halloumi slices.

Healthy Kitchen Hack: Can't find halloumi cheese in your store? Use cheese curds or string cheese (freeze the string cheese for 1 hour first) instead. Follow the coating

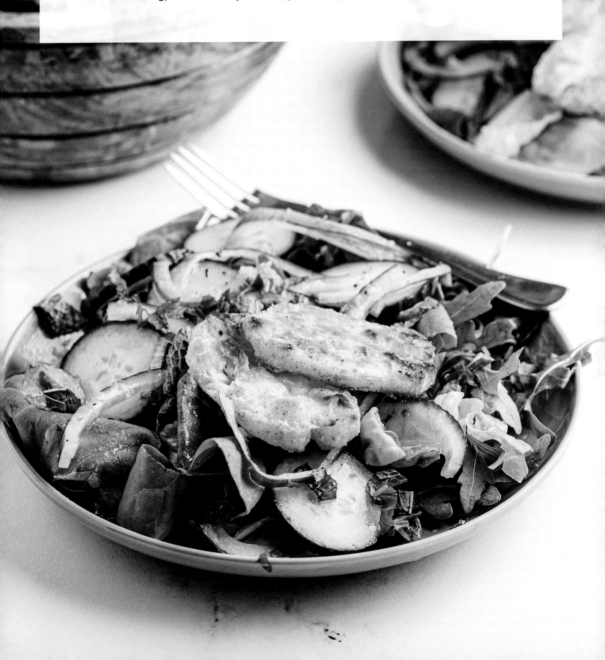

directions (brush lightly with water if the coating doesn't stick to frozen cheese) and then broil as directed above.

Per Serving: Calories: 283; Total Fat: 21g; Saturated Fat: 11g; Cholesterol: 50mg; Sodium: 669mg; Total Carbohydrates: 9g; Fiber: 3g; Protein: 14g

Grilled Greek Salad Skewers

SERVES 4
Prep time: 20 minutes
Cook time: 10 minutes

2 tablespoons extra-virgin olive oil

½ cup jarred or canned pitted black olives, drained and brine reserved

1 tablespoon red wine vinegar

1 teaspoon honey

¾ teaspoon dried oregano, divided

¼ teaspoon kosher or sea salt

¼ teaspoon black pepper

2 heads romaine lettuce, cut in half lengthwise

2 cups cherry or grape tomatoes

1 medium zucchini, cut into 1-inch pieces

1 medium red onion, cut into 1-inch wedges

½ cup chopped fresh mint or basil, leaves and stems

4 ounces feta cheese, crumbled

Much like roasting, grilling brings another layer of smoky, earthy, and slightly sweet flavor to just about any veggie, including lettuce! If you tried our "regrowing romaine" Hack on page 70, use your harvest in this recipe, which is best made at the peak of the summer zucchini and tomato season, naturally. You could skip the skewering and grilling altogether (see the Hack that follows this recipe), but we encourage you to try it this way at least once. It's a no-brainer when you're already firing up the grill for your main course!

Soak eight 10- or 12-inch (compostable) wooden skewers in warm water for 15 minutes or have metal skewers ready.

In a large bowl, whisk together the oil, 2 tablespoons of the olive brine, vinegar, honey, ½ teaspoon oregano, salt, and pepper. One by one, dredge the four romaine halves through the vinaigrette, turning each side to make sure they get fully seasoned. Slightly shake the excess dressing back into the bowl, place the dressed romaine halves on a plate, and set aside (there will still be a good amount of vinaigrette in the bowl).

In the same bowl with the vinaigrette, toss together the olives, tomatoes, zucchini, red onion, and mint until well incorporated. Thread the veggies onto the skewers, alternating items on each. (You may have enough ingredients for an extra skewer or two depending on which length you use.)

Coat the cold grill with cooking spray, then heat to 400°F, or medium-high heat. Place the skewers on the hot grill, cover, and grill until the veggies have grill marks and have softened, 7 to 8 minutes, turning them over halfway through that time. Transfer the skewers to a platter. Place the romaine halves, cut-side down, on the grill and grill, uncovered, until slightly charred, 1 to 2 minutes.

To serve, coarsely chop the charred romaine and divide among four salad bowls. Divide the feta cheese among the bowls and sprinkle with the remaining ¼ teaspoon oregano. Arrange two grilled vegetable kebabs on top of each salad bowl and serve immediately.

Healthy Kitchen Hack: When it comes to grilling, a gas grill is typically a better option over a charcoal grill. Gas is more energy-efficient as it takes much less time to heat up and produces few air pollutants. Get into the habit of cleaning your grill after every use to keep it working at its fullest energy-efficient potential (see Serena's cleaning Hack on page 200). If you don't have a grill or would rather cook inside, most grilling recipes are adaptable to stovetop cooking via a grill pan or skillet. Your oven broiler or toaster oven often are good options too— just keep a close eye on your food as cooking times will vary a bit.

Per Serving: Calories: 237; Total Fat: 16g; Saturated Fat: 6g; Cholesterol: 25mg; Sodium: 534mg; Total Carbohydrates: 19g; Fiber: 9g; Protein: 9g

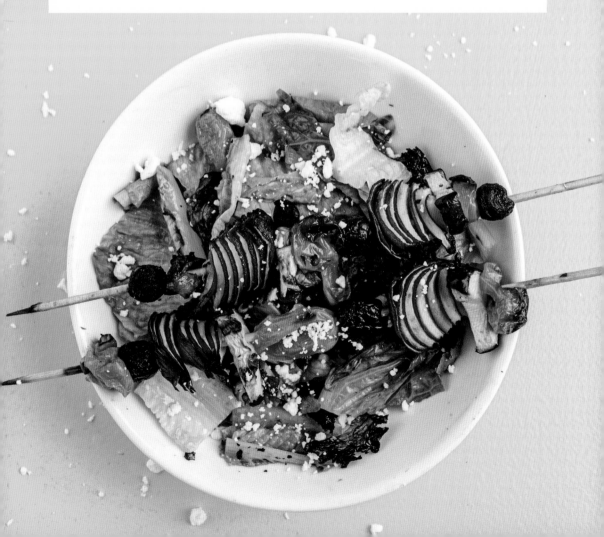

Spinach Salad with Balsamic Goat Cheese Dressing

SERVES 4
Prep time: 10 minutes

½ **cup softened, crumbled goat cheese (about 2 ounces)**

3 tablespoons balsamic vinegar

1 tablespoon extra-virgin olive oil

1 teaspoon honey

¼ **teaspoon kosher or sea salt**

¼ **teaspoon black pepper**

8 cups fresh baby or chopped spinach

1 cup chopped fresh parsley, cilantro, or basil (or a combination), leaves and stems

¼ **cup thinly sliced sweet onion**

¼ **cup pumpkin seeds or sunflower seeds**

2 cups fresh berries *or* ⅓ **cup dried cherries, dried cranberries, or dried blueberries**

Eating salad more often can be tricky because of the quick perishability of fresh produce. But this *is* a Mediterranean diet cookbook, after all, so we wanted to make eating more vibrant, veggie- and herb-filled salads super easy and inviting. And that's why we love offering up a bunch of yummy homemade dressing options. Our balsamic goat cheese drizzle is yet another quick one that's so good—and easy—you may even commit it to memory. We particularly like it tossed with spinach, but it works well with any leafy greens you prefer.

In a serving bowl, using a fork, mash the goat cheese into the vinegar, oil, honey, salt, and pepper, then whisk everything together, adding a little water if needed to reach a drizzling consistency.

Add the spinach, herbs, onion, and seeds and toss everything to coat. Add the berries and serve.

Healthy Kitchen Hack: Don't have goat cheese on hand for this dressing? No worries—all you truly need to dress a salad is the classic combo of oil and vinegar. Combine 2 parts olive oil to 1 part vinegar (any kind!) in a salad bowl; whisk together with salt and pepper and then taste to see if you'd like a splash more vinegar. You can also whisk in a little Dijon mustard to emulsify the dressing, if you wish. Then add your salad greens and other ingredients, toss, and serve.

Per Serving: Calories: 197; Total Fat: 12g; Saturated Fat: 3g; Cholesterol: 6mg; Sodium: 235mg; Total Carbohydrates: 19g; Fiber: 4g; Protein: 7g

Israeli Couscous "Pasta Salad"

SERVES 4
Prep time: 10 minutes
Cook time: 15 minutes

1 teaspoon extra-virgin olive oil

1 (8-ounce) box whole-wheat or regular Israeli couscous (about 1⅓ cups)

⅛ teaspoon kosher or sea salt

½ batch Honey, Orange, and Scallion Vinaigrette (page 70), plus the mandarin oranges from the can (reserved separately)

4 celery stalks and leaves, finely chopped

1 (2.25-ounce) can sliced black olives, drained (liquid saved for another use), *or* ½ cup sliced green olives

¼ cup shelled pistachios or walnut pieces

¼ teaspoon black pepper

Here's our Mediterranean twist on the classic picnic pasta salad that you can make year-round thanks to pantry staples. Take advantage of leftover Honey, Orange, and Scallion Vinaigrette (page 70) to stir up this recipe featuring Israeli couscous (or pearl couscous), which is similar in texture, taste, and size to tiny pasta shapes like pastina. For an extra layer of nuttiness, we give the couscous a quick toast in the pot before boiling. Serve this sunny orange and green dish warm or at room temperature for lunch or a light dinner. Or if you can be patient, chill it in the fridge to intensify all the ingredient flavors and to enjoy it at a cooler temperature—the traditional pasta salad way.

Heat the oil in a medium saucepan over medium heat. Add the couscous and cook, stirring frequently, until lightly brown, 3 to 4 minutes. Pour in 1¾ cups warm water and bring to a boil. Reduce the heat to medium-low, cover, and cook for 12 minutes or until the liquid is absorbed. Remove from the heat, mix in the salt, and transfer to a large serving bowl. Cool in the refrigerator for about 10 minutes (if serving the salad cold).

Remove the bowl from the refrigerator. Pour in the vinaigrette. Add the mandarin oranges, celery, olives, nuts, and pepper. Mix well and serve immediately, or cover and return to the refrigerator to chill longer. (If you're not serving the salad within 2 hours, mix all the ingredients together except the nuts, then stir them in right before serving.)

Healthy Kitchen Hack: To make a heartier, protein-packed pasta salad, mix in canned tuna, salmon, or smoked trout. Make it cheesy with some crumbled feta, crumbled Gorgonzola, or diced fresh mozzarella. Or keep it plant-based and toss in canned or cooked chickpeas, cannellini beans, or lentils.

Per Serving: Calories: 373; Total Fat: 13g; Saturated Fat: 2g; Cholesterol: 0mg; Sodium: 345mg; Total Carbohydrates: 57g; Fiber: 5g; Protein: 9g

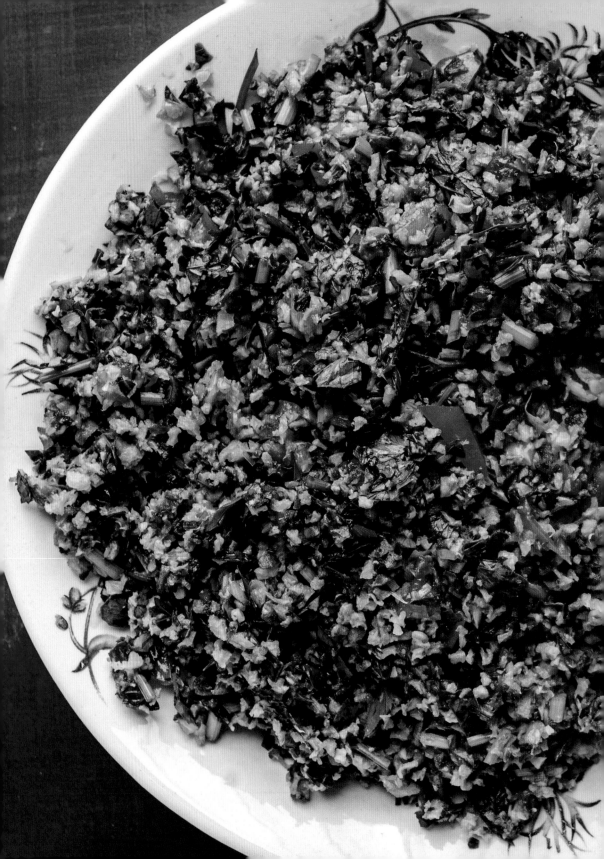

Sides

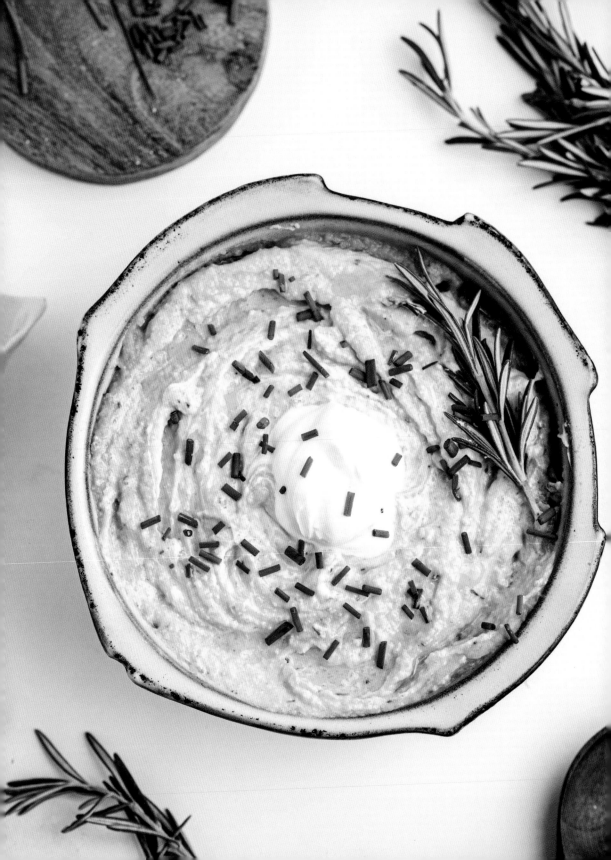

EGG-FREE, GLUTEN-FREE, NUT-FREE, VEGETARIAN

Rosemary and Chive Whipped Butternut Squash with Mascarpone Swirl

SERVES 6
Prep time: 10 minutes
Cook time: 15 minutes

1 (2½-pound) butternut squash

¼ cup plus 1 teaspoon 2% milk, divided

¼ cup minced fresh chives

1 tablespoon finely chopped fresh rosemary leaves *or* 1 teaspoon dried rosemary

1 tablespoon extra-virgin olive oil

½ teaspoon kosher or sea salt, divided

¼ teaspoon black pepper

1 lemon

3 tablespoons mascarpone cheese

Butternut squash is a darling of the fall season, with its sweet flavor and beautiful golden hue. We encourage you to buy it whole because it's less expensive, there's no extra packaging, *and* you get the seeds. But we get that it can be intimidating to chop up the whole thing, so we have a trick to make cutting it in half a breeze: soften the squash in the microwave! You can serve this whipped dish as an updated Thanksgiving side or as an anytime swap for your usual potato side dish. And of course, save those seeds for a roasted crunchy snack or to make our Toasted Squash Seeds and Cheese Board (page 61).

Using a sharp paring knife or a fork, make about 15 slits or holes around the entire squash to release steam during microwaving. Microwave the squash on a large microwave-safe plate on high for 5 minutes.

Using oven mitts, remove the squash and transfer to a cutting board. Holding the squash with an oven mitt, carefully cut it in half crosswise, then cut each half in half lengthwise (try to get four somewhat equal pieces). Scoop out the seeds and save for another use (if you're going to toast them, it's fine if some of the flesh is still attached to the seeds).

Place the four pieces on the microwave-safe plate, cut-side down, and cover with a microwave-safe bowl large enough to cover the squash. Microwave for 8 to 10 minutes, until the middle part of the pieces are cooked through and easily pierced with a fork (the heavier the squash, the longer it will take for all the flesh to soften).

Again, using oven mitts, remove the squash and carefully lift the bowl, being mindful of the steam escaping to avoid getting burned. Let cool for 5 to 10 minutes on a wire rack.

continued

Scoop the squash flesh into a blender or food processor. Add ¼ cup milk, the chives, rosemary, oil, ¼ teaspoon salt, and pepper. Puree until well blended.

Using a Microplane or citrus zester, grate the zest from the lemon over the blender. Cut the lemon in half; squeeze in 1 tablespoon lemon juice (save the remaining juice for another use). Puree again until well blended.

In a small bowl, whisk together the mascarpone cheese and remaining 1 teaspoon milk.

To serve, scoop the whipped squash into a shallow serving platter or bowl. Drizzle the mascarpone mix over the top, then use a butter knife to swirl it throughout the squash. Sprinkle the remaining ¼ teaspoon salt over the top and serve.

Healthy Kitchen Hack: For some recipe variations to this yummy side dish, swap in our Made-in-Minutes Homemade Ricotta **(page 48)** for the mascarpone cheese. Or add some heat and sweet by using a mix of smoked paprika and ground cinnamon instead of rosemary. If you have leftovers, reheat and mix the whipped squash into cooked grains or pasta as a sauce, serve as a dip with raw veggies and pita bread, or mix with broth and reheat as a butternut squash soup.

Per Serving: Calories: 114; Total Fat: 6g; Saturated Fat: 2g; Cholesterol: 11mg; Sodium: 174mg; Total Carbohydrates: 16g; Fiber: 5g; Protein: 2g

"My whole family (including our dog, Mushroom) loved this dish! Extra bonus: I used the leftovers to make a yummy butternut squash soup in minutes for lunch the next day."

—Jessica from Silver Spring, MD

Smashed Potatoes with Romesco Sauce

SERVES 6
Prep time: 10 minutes
Cook time: 20 minutes

1½ pounds yellow baby or small red potatoes

¾ teaspoon kosher or sea salt, divided

1 (12-ounce) jar roasted red peppers, drained
Save the liquid! See Hack

1 (14.5-ounce) can regular or fire-roasted diced tomatoes

2 garlic cloves, peeled

2 teaspoons red wine vinegar

1 teaspoon smoked paprika

¼ teaspoon black pepper

3 tablespoons extra-virgin olive oil, divided

½ cup torn, stale bread or toast

3 tablespoons shaved Manchego or Parmesan cheese

1 tablespoon fresh thyme leaves, plus more for serving

We've upgraded the same old potato side with this fun and super yummy dish. Typically, smashed potato recipes call for boiling them and then roasting for at least 20 minutes. But here, we fire up the broiler to cut the oven cooking time down to mere minutes. Though you'll need only half of the smoky, super-easy-to-whip-up Spanish romesco sauce for these potatoes, practicality is our middle name and we'll help you use it up. You can use the other half in our Spanish Broccoli-Stuffed Calzones (page 131) or as a delicious alternative pasta sauce. You could also freeze the remainder of the sauce in an ice cube tray to use as 1-tablespoon "flavor bombs" for future soup or chili recipes.

Put the potatoes in a large pot and fill with water to about an inch over the potatoes. Add ¼ teaspoon salt, cover, and bring to a boil. Uncover, reduce the heat to medium, and cook until just fork-tender, 12 to 15 minutes. Drain the potatoes in a colander, then return them to the pot.

While the potatoes cook, make the romesco sauce. In a blender or food processor, combine the drained roasted red peppers, tomatoes with their juices, garlic, vinegar, smoked paprika, ¼ teaspoon salt, and the black pepper. Puree the ingredients, then slowly drizzle in 2 tablespoons oil while the blender runs. Add the bread, then continue to process until the sauce is smooth. Reserve half of the sauce for the potatoes and save the remaining sauce for another recipe.

Arrange the top oven rack about 4 inches under the broiler. Preheat the broiler to high. Spray a large rimmed baking sheet with cooking spray.

Using a fork or tongs, one by one, transfer the hot potatoes to the prepared baking sheet. Using the bottom of a small glass, press down and smash each potato so they are the same thickness. Drizzle the smashed

continued

potatoes with the remaining 1 tablespoon oil and sprinkle with the shaved cheese and fresh thyme. Broil for 3 to 4 minutes, depending on how crispy you like your potatoes. Remove from the oven.

Sprinkle the potatoes with the remaining ¼ teaspoon salt and more fresh thyme if desired. Spoon some of the reserved romesco sauce over each potato and serve warm, right on the baking sheet, with the remaining sauce in a bowl alongside.

Healthy Kitchen Hack: We used to toss out the jarred roasted red pepper liquid until we changed our mindset to repurpose more byproducts in the kitchen. These peppers are often preserved in a brine of water, salt, and citric acid (or less commonly in olive oil). As it takes on some red pepper flavor, that brine is a fine addition to other recipes. Store the liquid back in the jar in your refrigerator (for up to 2 weeks) for future recipes. Mix it with broth for vegetable-based soups or combine it with water when cooking pasta or other grains. Or, when making those Spanish Broccoli-Stuffed Calzones (page 131), brush the dough with the pepper liquid before baking to get a lovely golden hue and an extra hint of flavor.

Per Serving: Calories: 157; Total Fat: 6g; Saturated Fat: 1g; Cholesterol: 2mg; Sodium: 366mg; Total Carbohydrates: 24g; Fiber: 3g; Protein: 4g

"I loved the sauce and can't wait to use it in other recipes. We will definitely be having this delicious dish again!"

—Jen from Boston, MA

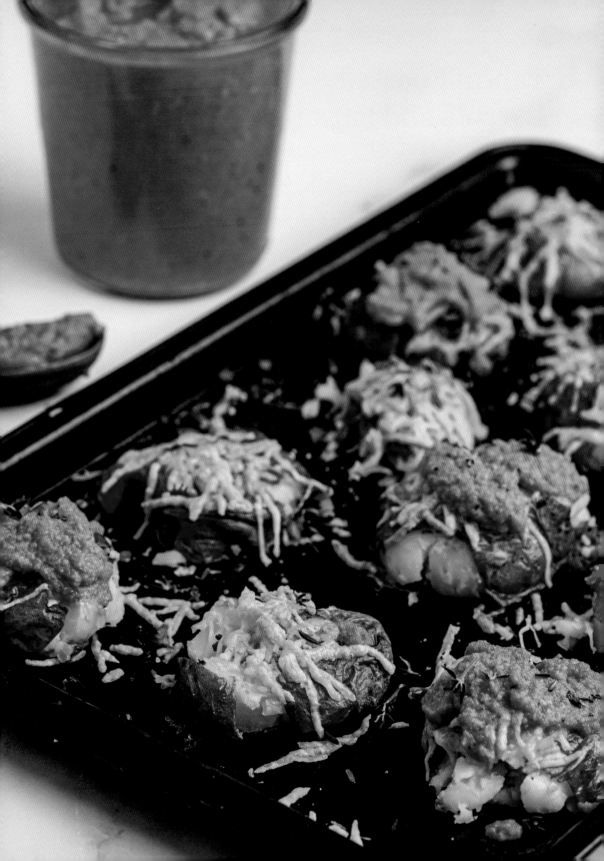

Tahini Roasted Carrots and Parsnips

SERVES 6

Prep time: 10 minutes
Cook time: 30 minutes

1 lemon

2 tablespoons tahini

2 tablespoons extra-virgin olive oil

½ teaspoon kosher or sea salt

¼ teaspoon black pepper, divided

1 pound carrots, rinsed and scrubbed (see Hack)

1 pound parsnips, rinsed and scrubbed (see Hack)

2 teaspoons sesame seeds (optional)

Serena may or may not have told her children that the parsnips in this dish were "yellow carrots." When her eldest became savvy enough to announce the correct title of the golden veggies as parsnips, Serena got another surprise from her youngest, who replied, "Mom, I actually like the parsnips better than the carrots—they're sweeter." Enjoy this sweet and savory dish from late fall through early spring, during the root veggies' peak season.

Preheat the oven to 450°F. Line a large rimmed baking sheet with parchment paper.

Using a Microplane or citrus zester, grate the zest from the lemon into a large bowl. Cut the lemon in half and squeeze 2 tablespoons juice into the bowl. (Reserve the remaining juice for serving.) Whisk in the tahini, oil, salt, and pepper. Set aside.

Slice the carrots and parsnips in half lengthwise, cut each half into 3-inch pieces, so that all the chunks are roughly the same thickness (if a chunk is too thick, cut it in half lengthwise). Toss the carrots and parsnips in the bowl with the tahini mixture until well coated.

Spread out the vegetables evenly on the prepared baking sheet and drizzle with any tahini mixture remaining in the bowl. Roast for 25 to 30 minutes, until the vegetables are fork-tender.

If using sesame seeds, toast in a small skillet over medium heat, shaking occasionally, until the seeds start to turn golden and smell fragrant, 2 to 4 minutes.

Transfer the roasted vegetables to a serving dish and sprinkle with the sesame seeds, if using. Squeeze about 1 tablespoon lemon juice from the remaining lemon half over the veggies and serve.

Healthy Kitchen Hack: Leaving the peels on carrots, parsnips, beets, potatoes, and other root vegetables keeps in the best nutrition since the most potent antioxidants are located just beneath the skin. Not to mention, it also cuts back on food waste. To get these veggies clean, soak them in cold water for 1 to 2 minutes to soften any dirt, then scrub well with a vegetable brush under running water. But, whenever you do need to peel, you can still cut down on waste by stashing the scraps in the freezer and using them in our Veggie Scraps Broth recipe on page 120.

Per Serving: Calories: 165; Total Fat: 8g; Saturated Fat: 1g; Cholesterol: 0mg; Sodium: 225mg; Total Carbohydrates: 23g; Fiber: 7g; Protein: 3g

Toasted Cauliflower Tabbouleh

SERVES 4
Prep time: 5 minutes
Cook time: 30 minutes

4 tablespoons extra-virgin olive oil, divided

1 (10-ounce) package frozen riced cauliflower

½ teaspoon kosher or sea salt, divided

1 lemon

1 garlic clove, minced

½ teaspoon black pepper

2 cups chopped fresh tomatoes, or canned and drained diced tomatoes

2 cups chopped fresh parsley, leaves and stems

1 cup chopped fresh mint, leaves and stems

"We loved how zesty and light this salad was. We were also surprised how good 2 whole cups of parsley can be! It was great to pack in my husband's lunches."

—Sarah from Maryville, IL

Frozen veggies are sustainable, nutritious, affordable, and super convenient because they come precut, but when boiled or steamed, they can be a bit soft and lacking in flavor. Here's our favorite way to make them taste terrific: roast them in a really hot oven with a good amount of oil. Roasting this way gives a bold, toasted flavor and great texture to any frozen vegetables, such as broccoli, carrots, corn, peppers, and even riced cauliflower, which we use in this dish! The toasted cauliflower stands in for nutty wheat bulgur in this classic Mediterranean salad of bright fresh parsley and mint, juicy tomatoes, and tart lemon, for some of the best tabbouleh you've tasted. (Save any leftovers to make our Spicy Fish Shawarma Bowls on page 225.)

Pour 2 tablespoons oil on a large rimmed baking sheet and put it in the oven. Preheat the oven to 450°F (with the sheet inside).

In a large serving bowl, toss together the frozen cauliflower and 1 tablespoon oil until well coated. Carefully remove the hot baking sheet from the oven and spread the cauliflower out in a thin layer; bake for 10 minutes. Carefully remove the hot baking sheet and stir; spread the cauliflower into a thin layer again and bake for an additional 10 minutes. Once more, remove the pan, stir, and return to the oven to cook for an additional 8 to 10 minutes, until the cauliflower is dark golden brown. Remove from the oven and sprinkle with ¼ teaspoon salt; toss well. Cool completely (you can speed this up by scraping onto a plate and stirring a few times).

While the cauliflower roasts, using a Microplane or citrus zester, grate the zest from the lemon into the now-empty bowl; cut the lemon in half and squeeze in 2 to 3 tablespoons lemon juice. Add the garlic and let sit for at least 15 minutes to mellow the raw garlic.

While the cauliflower cools, to the lemon garlic mixture, add the remaining 1 tablespoon oil, remaining ¼ teaspoon salt, and the pepper; whisk to combine. Add the tomatoes, parsley, and mint, toss to combine, and serve.

Healthy Kitchen Hack: While roasting frozen riced cauliflower makes this recipe really good, if you are short on time, microwaving the cauliflower in minutes also makes for a delicious bowl of tabbouleh. Simply follow the microwave cooking directions on the package and drain well, then follow the recipe instructions here for the remaining ingredients. And when you pick up that bag of riced cauliflower at the store, grab a few more as they last for months in the freezer. They can seamlessly add vegetable nutrition to a bowl of plain rice and many more meals from scrambled eggs to canned soups to baked pasta.

Per Serving: Calories: 169; Total Fat: 15g; Saturated Fat: 2g; Cholesterol: 0mg; Sodium: 280mg; Total Carbohydrates: 10g; Fiber: 4g; Protein: 3g

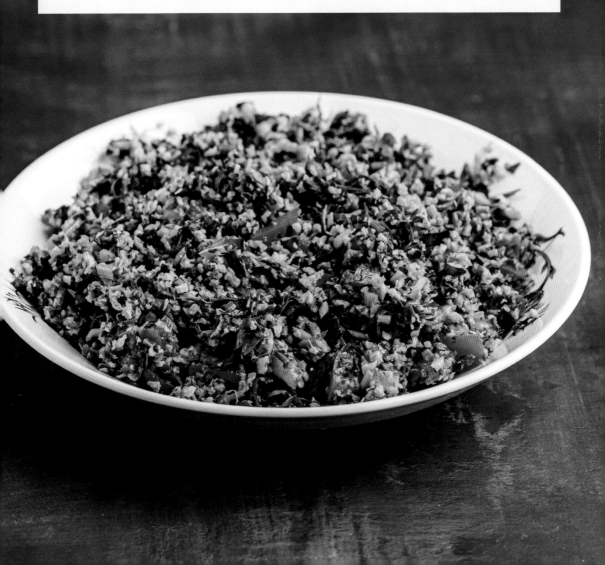

Roasted Harissa Zucchini Spears

SERVES 6
Prep time: 10 minutes
Cook time: 20 minutes

2 medium or 1 large
zucchini

1 lime

1 tablespoon sweet
paprika

1½ teaspoons ground
cumin

½ teaspoon ground
coriander

¼–½ teaspoon smoked
paprika

¼ teaspoon garlic
powder

¼ teaspoon kosher or
sea salt

¼ teaspoon black
pepper

2 tablespoons extra-
virgin olive oil

¼ cup finely chopped
fresh mint, leaves and
stems

2 tablespoons finely
chopped fresh chives
or scallions (green
onions), green and
white parts
*Save the stem roots!
See page 70*

Turn to this zesty veggie side when you're swimming in zucchini during those summer months. The homemade harissa seasoning from our Harissa-Spiced Chicken Kebabs (page 249) is equally delectable on any summer squash. We like to make this dish after we've already heated up the oven for another recipe and bake two sheets at the same time to cut down on oven time. For more energy efficiency tips, see our alternative cooking methods in the Healthy Kitchen Hack.

Arrange the oven racks to the upper-middle and lower-middle positions. Preheat the oven to 450°F. Set wire racks in two large rimmed baking sheets.

Trim the ends of the zucchini (and add to your freezer bag for our Veggie Scraps Broth recipe on page 120). Cut each zucchini in half crosswise (if using one large zucchini, cut it crosswise into three sections). Cut each section in half lengthwise, then cut into spears that are ¾ to 1 inch wide.

Using a Microplane or citrus zester, grate the zest from the lime over a large bowl; cut the lime in half and squeeze in the juice. Add the sweet paprika, cumin, coriander, smoked paprika, garlic powder, salt, pepper, and oil; whisk to combine. Add the zucchini spears and, using your hands, gently toss to coat until all the spears are thoroughly covered with the harissa paste.

Line up the spears on the two wire racks, making sure they are not touching. Bake for 10 minutes, then switch the top sheet to the bottom rack and vice versa. Bake for an additional 10 to 12 minutes, until the spears are cooked through to your preference. Let cool for 5 to 10 minutes, then transfer to a serving platter and sprinkle with the mint and chives. Serve immediately.

Healthy Kitchen Hack: For those extra hot days, avoid heating up your kitchen with the oven and cook these spears on the outside grill, in your toaster oven, or in an air fryer. Check on them after about 5 minutes and every few minutes after.

Per Serving: Calories: 67; Total Fat: 5g; Saturated Fat: 108g; Cholesterol: 0mg; Sodium: 108mg; Total Carbohydrates: 5g; Fiber: 2g; Protein: 2g

Honey and Salt Roasted Brussels Sprouts

SERVES 4
Prep time: 10 minutes
Cook time: 15 minutes

1 pound Brussels sprouts, halved

1½ tablespoons extra-virgin olive oil

¼ teaspoon kosher or sea salt

¼ teaspoon black pepper

1 tablespoon balsamic vinegar

1 tablespoon honey

¼ cup sunflower seeds, pepitas, pistachios, walnuts, and/or other nuts or seeds

¼ cup dried cherries, cranberries, raisins, chopped dried apricots, chopped dried figs, and/or other dried fruit

These Brussels sprouts are beautifully foolproof, wonderfully flexible, and almost guaranteed to get requests for seconds from everyone at the table. Start with the sprouts (or sub in broccoli or cauliflower florets), then (1) drizzle with olive oil, (2) roast, (3) sweeten with balsamic vinegar and honey, and (4) add some seeds/nuts and dried fruits—and you've got one delish side dish with dozens of flavor combinations you can create from one basic recipe. Eat warm straight from the baking sheet, serve at room temperature, or eat cold the next day for lunch with a hearty whole grain to make it a meal.

Preheat the oven to 425°F.

On a large rimmed baking sheet, toss together the Brussels sprouts and oil with your hands until evenly coated. Sprinkle with the salt and pepper. Arrange all the sprouts so they are cut-side down on the sheet. Bake for about 15 minutes, until the cut sides are dark brown. Carefully remove the sheet from the oven and drizzle with the vinegar and honey; toss to coat. Sprinkle the sprouts with the seeds and/or nuts. Return to the oven for about 5 minutes, until the seeds/nuts are toasted and the honey has glazed the sprouts. Add the dried fruit, mix well, and serve from the baking sheet.

Healthy Kitchen Hack: Just as in our Toasted Cauliflower Tabbouleh (page 96), you can roast vegetables straight from frozen, no need to thaw. This tasty dish can be made at a moment's notice when you have a well-stocked freezer—and frozen veggies are often more budget-friendly than fresh. Toss 12 to 16 ounces frozen whole Brussels sprouts in oil as directed and then roast for 25 minutes, until they are heated through and dark brown on the bottom; if not, stir and roast for about 10 minutes more. Then follow the recipe instructions.

Per Serving: Calories: 196; Total Fat: 10g; Saturated Fat: 1g; Cholesterol: 0mg; Sodium: 151mg; Total Carbohydrates: 25g; Fiber: 6g; Protein: 6g

Lemon Charred Asparagus with Zesty Garlic Sauce

SERVES 4
Prep time: 10 minutes
Cook time: 15 minutes

1 (2-ounce) tin anchovies in olive oil, undrained

3 tablespoons extra-virgin olive oil, divided

2 garlic cloves, minced

2 lemons

1 pound asparagus, trimmed (see Hack)

¼ teaspoon kosher or sea salt

¼ teaspoon black pepper

1 cup plain 2% Greek yogurt

2 tablespoons chopped fresh chives

In our humble opinion, broiling makes vegetables (and lemons!) irresistible. (But keep a sharp eye out—Deanna has had many unsuccessful rounds with her broiler over the years after getting distracted for mere seconds in the kitchen.) Turn to this recipe in the spring when the first asparagus hits your market or pops up in your garden. Topping this asparagus is a zesty garlic sauce that unexpectedly became one of Deanna's favorite flavors in the entire cookbook. Imagine a drizzle-able version of sour cream and onion dip, but made with yogurt, garlic, and a surprise ingredient your family or guests might never guess, even when tasting this magical sauce.

Arrange the top oven rack about 4 inches under the broiler. Preheat the broiler to high.

Using a fork, remove 6 anchovies from the tin and set aside (save the remaining anchovies in the tin for another use). In a small saucepan, heat 2 tablespoons olive oil and all the oil from the anchovy tin over medium heat. Add the garlic and cook, stirring constantly, for about 30 seconds. Reduce the heat to medium-low and add the anchovies; mash them up with the back of a spoon or spatula while stirring frequently for 1 minute. Continue to cook, stirring occasionally, for a total cooking time of 10 minutes. Pour the garlic-anchovy mixture into a small bowl and set aside to cool for about 5 minutes.

While the garlic and anchovies cook, using a Microplane or citrus zester, grate the zest from the lemons into a small bowl. Cut each lemon into 8 or 10 slices and set aside.

Put the asparagus spears on a large rimmed baking sheet. Drizzle with the remaining 1 tablespoon olive oil and sprinkle with the salt and pepper. Using your hands, mix the spears until well coated, then push them to one side of the sheet. Scatter the lemon slices all over the now-oiled baking sheet, then arrange the asparagus on top of them. Sprinkle the asparagus with half of the reserved lemon zest.

Broil the asparagus for 3 minutes, then use tongs or a fork to turn over the spears and broil for an additional 2 to 3 minutes or until the asparagus is blistered on both sides and tender. Transfer the asparagus to a serving tray, along with the charred lemon slices.

While the asparagus cooks, add the yogurt and 3 tablespoons water to the bowl with the garlic-anchovy oil. Whisk until a drizzle-like consistency forms, adding extra water if needed, 1 tablespoon at a time.

To serve, drizzle the asparagus and lemons with half of the yogurt sauce (store the remaining sauce in a jar in the refrigerator for up to 4 days and use it on any vegetable or salad). Sprinkle the asparagus and lemons with the chives and the remaining lemon zest and serve.

Healthy Kitchen Hack: For many years, we diligently used the "bend until it snaps" method for getting rid of the wooden ends of asparagus spears, but it turns out we were wasting a good-size edible portion of the veggies. The better (and faster) way? Simply cut off any white-gray ends, which should be no more than an inch in length. And unless the recipe has you finely chopping up the asparagus (like in our Whole Leek and Asparagus Soup on page 106), toss those white ends into your freezer Veggie Scraps bag (see page 120 for our Veggie Scraps Broth recipe), and from now on, enjoy even *more* of the asparagus in your favorite recipes.

Per Serving: Calories: 131; Total Fat: 10g; Saturated Fat: 2g; Cholesterol: 10mg; Sodium: 485mg; Total Carbohydrates: 6g; Fiber: 3g; Protein: 7g

Crispy Parmesan Green Beans

SERVES 4
Prep time: 10 minutes
Cook time: 15 minutes

⅓ cup panko bread crumbs

¼ cup grated Parmesan cheese

¼ teaspoon kosher or sea salt

¼ teaspoon black pepper

⅛–¼ teaspoon crushed red pepper

⅓ cup plain 2% Greek yogurt

1 pound green beans, trimmed

1 lemon

Deanna thought her favorite way to eat her less-than-favorite green beans was to char them under the broiler, but this preparation has completely changed her mind. You won't believe that a recipe this simple can make basic vegetables become so irresistible! The key to creating a coating that will stick to veggies (and fish and chicken, too) is to add some type of "glue" before the breading. Often a beaten egg is used, but we also like using Greek yogurt thinned with a little water for that tangy Mediterranean flavor. Switch up the flavor by adding different spices to the coating, like za'atar, smoked paprika, sesame seeds, or any dried herb.

Arrange the oven racks to the upper-middle and lower-middle positions. Preheat the oven to 425°F. Coat two large rimmed baking sheets with cooking spray.

In a large bowl, whisk together the panko, Parmesan cheese, salt, black pepper, and crushed red pepper.

In a large bowl, whisk together the yogurt and 2 tablespoons water. To ensure evenly distributed coating, add half of the green beans at a time and gently toss, using your hands, until all the beans are coated. Transfer the beans to the panko coating and again use your hands to gently toss until all the beans are breaded. Spread out the beans on one of the prepared baking sheets. Repeat the process with the remaining beans, spreading them out on the other sheet.

Bake for 8 minutes, then switch the top tray to the bottom rack and vice versa. Bake for an additional 3 to 5 minutes, until the beans are cooked through to your preference. Transfer the beans to a serving platter. Using a Microplane or citrus zester, grate the zest from the lemon over the green beans. Cut the lemon into wedges and serve alongside.

Healthy Kitchen Hack: Though not technically a Mediterranean staple, panko bread crumbs are our go-to ingredient for any coating thanks to their flaky texture, which makes breaded foods taste lighter and crispier. But if you don't have panko on hand, you can swap in cornmeal, dried bread crumbs, or even crushed cornflakes. Or better yet, make your own bread crumbs with any stale bread (from sliced bread to pita) by toasting it in a toaster, toaster oven, or on a baking sheet in a 400°F oven (while you have the oven on for another recipe, to save energy). Cool the toasted bread and then blitz it in a food processor or blender until fine crumbs form. Store in a freezer-safe container in the freezer for up to 1 month.

Per Serving: Calories: 106; Total Fat: 2g; Saturated Fat: 1g; Cholesterol: 7mg; Sodium: 260mg; Total Carbohydrates: 16g; Fiber: 3g; Protein: 7g

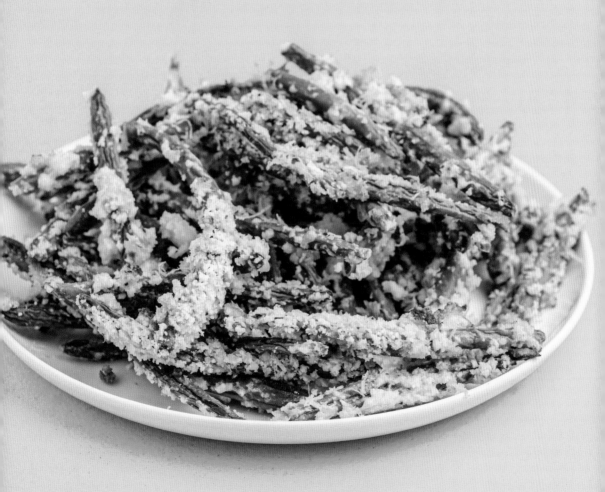

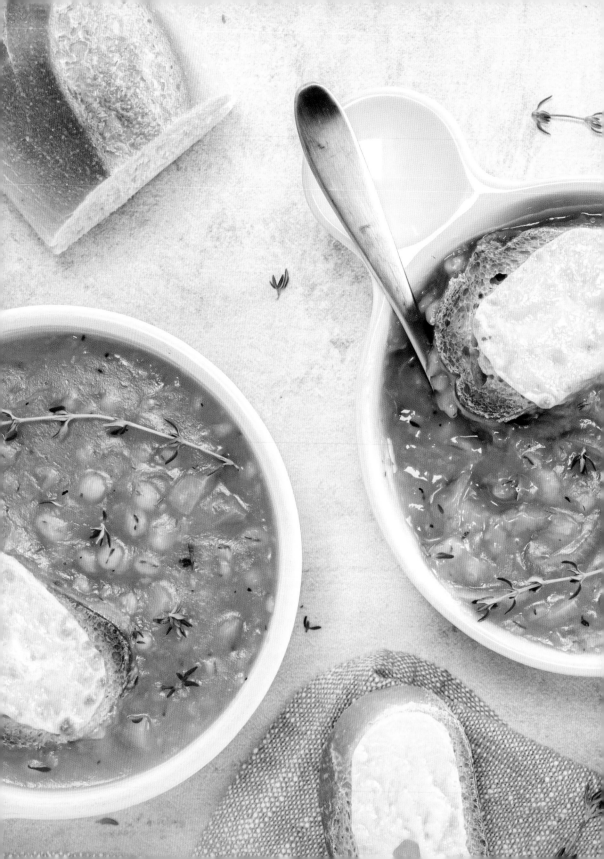

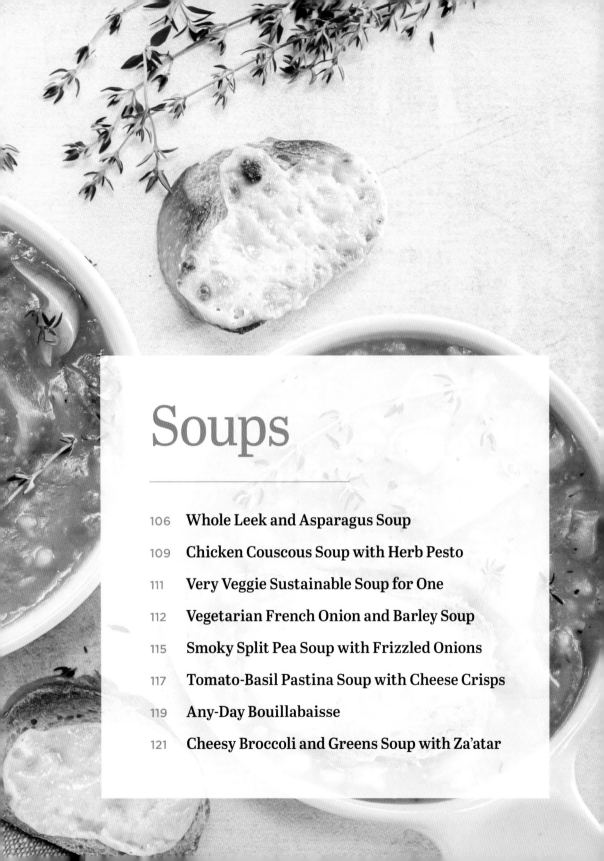

Soups

Whole Leek and Asparagus Soup

SERVES 6
Prep time: 15 minutes
Cook time: 30 minutes

1 pound asparagus
spears

1 leek

2 tablespoons extra-
virgin olive oil

1 lemon

3 tablespoons whole-
wheat flour

¼ teaspoon kosher or
sea salt

¼ teaspoon crushed
red pepper

4 cups Veggie Scraps
Broth (page 120) or
low-sodium vegetable
broth

½ cup shaved Asiago
or Parmesan cheese
(about 2 ounces)

Here's an easy "reduce food waste" fun fact: you *can* eat the
woody stems at the ends of asparagus—especially if you are
going to puree them into a soup or sauce. The trick is to give
them a head start in cook time over the more tender parts
of the spear. Ditto for the tougher dark green tops of leeks;
they are also totally edible and become buttery with a bit
more time in the pan. This springtime soup makes a star of
both asparagus and leeks, and we think you'll be blown away
by how flavorful this simple list of ingredients can be once it
makes it to your bowl.

Line up the asparagus spears on a cutting board and cut
off the tough ends from the tender stalks. Finely chop the
tough ends and then coarsely chop the remaining tender
stalks; keep the ends and stalks separate.

Cut the leek in half lengthwise. Rinse thoroughly to
remove any sandy grit. Finely chop the tough, dark green
ends, then thinly slice the tender, light green and white
ends. Keep the chopped dark green ends separate from
the light green and white slices.

Heat the oil in a large stockpot over medium
heat. Add the chopped tough asparagus stems and
the chopped dark green portions of the leek. Cook,
stirring occasionally, for 10 minutes. Add the remaining
asparagus, leek, and 2 tablespoons water, cover, and
cook for an additional 5 minutes.

While the vegetables cook, using a Microplane or
citrus zester, grate the zest from the lemon into a medium
bowl (reserve the lemon for finishing the soup). Add the
flour, salt, and crushed red pepper and stir.

Whisk the flour mixture into the asparagus and leeks
and cook for 1 minute, stirring frequently. Pour in the
broth, scrape up the brown bits on the bottom of the
pot, and bring to a boil. Turn the heat to medium-low
and cook for 20 minutes, stirring occasionally, until the
vegetables are tender. Turn off the heat.

With an immersion blender, puree the soup. (If using
a regular blender, carefully puree the mixture in batches
and then return it to the pot to warm before serving.)

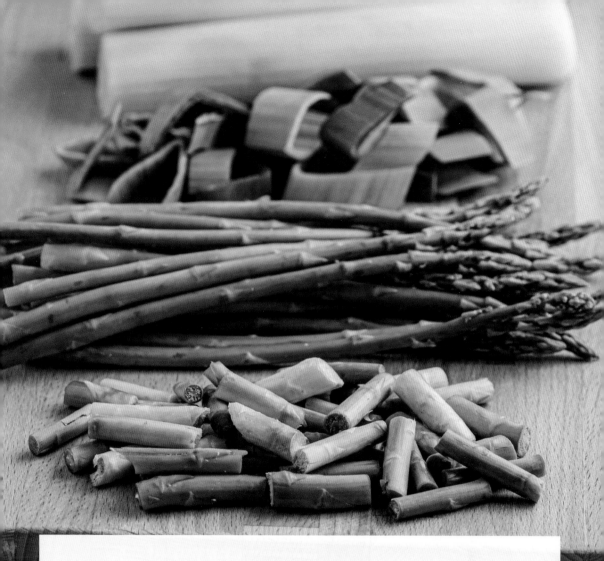

Cut the reserved lemon in half; squeeze about 2 tablespoons lemon juice into the soup and mix it in. Serve the cheese in a small bowl alongside the soup to use as a topping.

Healthy Kitchen Hack: What else can you do with those woody asparagus ends and the tough, dark green part of leeks? Puree fully cooked asparagus ends and mix into stews, pesto, and salad dressings. Use those cooked leek ends in any recipe as you would use sautéed onions, like a sauce for chicken, a base for pasta sauce, or a topping for pizza.

Per Serving: Calories: 127; **Total Fat:** 8g; **Saturated Fat:** 2g; **Cholesterol:** 7mg; **Sodium:** 332mg; **Total Carbohydrates:** 10g; **Fiber:** 3g; **Protein:** 6g

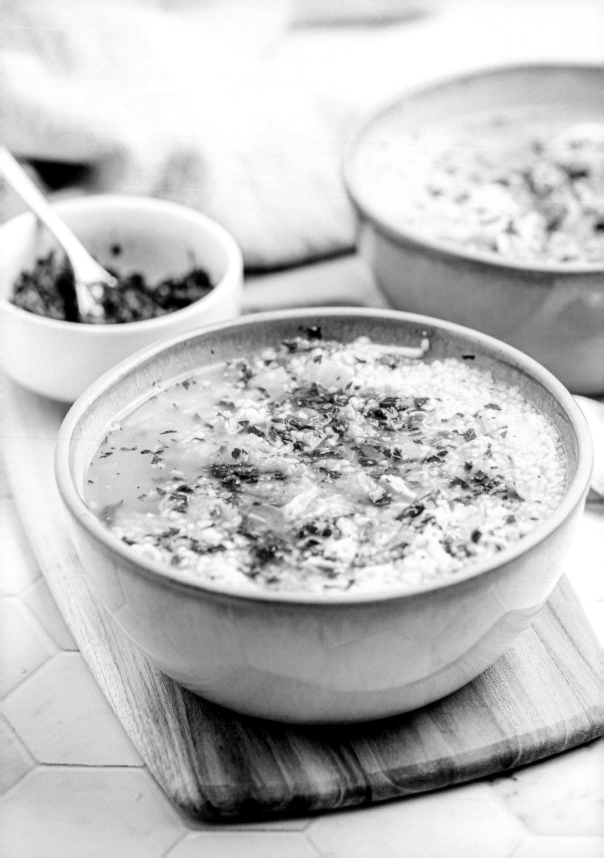

Chicken Couscous Soup with Herb Pesto

SERVES 6
Prep time: 15 minutes
Cook time: 30 minutes

2 (1-pound) frozen (or fresh—see Hack) boneless, skinless chicken breasts

1 medium onion (any type), chopped

¾ teaspoon kosher or sea salt, divided

1 garlic clove

1 lemon

2 cups chopped fresh herbs of choice, leaves and stems

1 tablespoon extra-virgin olive oil

1 (10-ounce) box couscous (*or* 1½ cups dry couscous)

Most cultures around the world find comfort in a bowl of chicken soup, and it is no different in the Mediterranean—but the exact ingredients and flavors change from region to region. In Morocco, chicken soup is traditionally made with tender couscous and is quite spicy. Instead of extra heat, we opted to season our version with a fresh lemony pesto to add a bold dose of antioxidants, while giving you another recipe to use up those fresh herbs like cilantro, parsley, basil, and/or mint. As for any leftovers, don't be surprised if you have to add a cup or two of water to the hearty soup when reheating as the couscous will absorb even more liquid in the fridge overnight.

In a large pot or Dutch oven over medium-high heat, combine the frozen chicken, 8 cups water, onion, and ½ teaspoon salt and bring to a gentle boil, then immediately turn the chicken pieces over with tongs. Cover the pot and remove from the heat. Allow the chicken to poach off the heat for 10 to 15 minutes (depending on the thickness of the breast) or until a meat thermometer inserted into the thickest part registers 155°F (the temperature will continue to rise while resting to reach the desired 165°F). Transfer the chicken to a cutting board to cool for about 5 minutes, reserving the pot with the onion and cooking water. Shred the chicken using two forks and set aside.

While the chicken cooks, make the pesto. Using the small holes on a box grater or a Microplane, grate the garlic into a medium serving bowl. Grate the zest from one lemon, add half of it into the bowl, and set the rest aside to finish off the recipe, then cut the lemon in half. Squeeze the juice of one half of the lemon into the bowl and add the herbs, oil, and remaining ¼ teaspoon salt. Mix well to incorporate all the ingredients.

Return the uncovered pot with the onion and cooking water to the stove and bring to a boil over high heat. Stir

continued

Chicken Couscous Soup with Herb Pesto *(continued)*

in the couscous. Cover, remove from the heat, and allow the couscous to hydrate for 5 minutes. Stir in the shredded chicken.

When ready to serve, squeeze the remaining half of the lemon into the soup. Serve the pesto alongside the soup as a topping, with remaining lemon zest on top if desired.

Healthy Kitchen Hack: You have a surprisingly sustainable friend in the freezer section: frozen chicken breasts. A family-sized bag (usually 2½, 5, or 10 pounds) is "fresh frozen," so the pieces remain tender and juicy in the freezer. High-quality chicken is frozen with a thin layer of ice to allow for extended shelf life for up to a year. For added convenience, in some recipes, frozen chicken can go straight from the freezer to the cooking pot, saving the thawing step, as we do with this soup. That said, if you are using thawed or fresh chicken breasts in this recipe, simply decrease the time that the chicken poaches in the pot by about 5 minutes.

Per Serving: Calories: 290; Total Fat 5g; Saturated Fat: 1g; Cholesterol: 55mg; Sodium: 281mg; Total Carbohydrates: 37g; Fiber: 3g; Protein: 23g

DAIRY-FREE, EGG-FREE, GLUTEN-FREE, NUT-FREE, VEGAN

Very Veggie Sustainable Soup for One

SERVES 1
Prep time: 5 minutes
Cook time: 5 minutes

1½ cups fresh or canned tomatoes (diced or crushed with their juices), divided

¼ cup chopped raw vegetables of choice (see headnote)

1 garlic clove, minced

1 teaspoon dried oregano

¼ teaspoon black pepper

¼ cup hummus or canned beans, drained, rinsed, and mashed

½ cup frozen vegetables or canned beans, drained and rinsed

¼ cup chopped fresh parsley, cilantro, or basil, leaves and stems

1 teaspoon extra-virgin olive oil

Soup warms the soul—and it just might help save the Earth. If we all made more soup, we'd probably have less food waste! Soup is a simple, smart, and satisfying way to use up those dibs and dabs of fresh vegetables hanging out in the refrigerator (such as carrots, celery, broccoli, zucchini, green beans, and/or cabbage) and almost magically turn them into a comforting meal—and this "kitchen sink" recipe is a blueprint to do just that. Serena's kids often make their own bowls of soup on Sunday nights when the family cleans out the fridge of leftovers before the new week begins.

In a large microwave-safe bowl, combine ½ cup tomatoes with their juices, chopped raw vegetables, garlic, oregano, and pepper and microwave on high for 2 minutes. Stir in the hummus (or mashed beans) until incorporated. Add the frozen vegetables (or beans) and microwave on high for 1 minute. Check the vegetables for doneness to your liking; we like our frozen vegetables just barely cooked, but if you like softer veggies, microwave for another 30 seconds to 1 minute. Stir in the remaining tomatoes with juices and microwave on high for 1 minute. Stir in the parsley, drizzle with oil, and enjoy straight from the large bowl—no need to dirty another dish!

Healthy Kitchen Hack: Think of this recipe as more of a template. Start with any leftover tomato product: besides diced or crushed tomatoes, you can use canned whole tomatoes, 1 cup tomato or pasta sauce, ½ cup tomato/vegetable juice, or ¼ cup tomato paste (just dilute it with enough water to make 1½ cups tomato liquid, which helps keep the sodium levels lower). Experiment with adding other leftover bits of fresh, canned, jarred, and/or frozen veggies. To make the soup for more than one, simply increase the measurements in the ingredient list per person accordingly; the cooking times will increase slightly.

Per Serving (using ¼ cup zucchini, ¼ cup canned black beans, ½ cup frozen corn/green bean/carrot mix): Calories: 221; Total Fat: 6g; Saturated Fat: 0g; Cholesterol: 0mg; Sodium: 580mg; Total Carbohydrates: 38g; Fiber: 16g; Protein: 10g

Vegetarian French Onion and Barley Soup

SERVES 8
Prep time: 15 minutes
Cook time: 4 hours

2 tablespoons extra-virgin olive oil

4 medium onions (any type), thinly sliced

1 cup uncooked pearl barley

8 cups Veggie Scraps Broth (page 120), low-sodium vegetable broth, or water

¼ cup dry red wine or red wine vinegar

2 tablespoons less-sodium soy sauce

1 tablespoon fresh thyme, leaves and stems, *or* 1 teaspoon dried thyme, plus sprigs for garnish if desired

1 bay leaf

¼ teaspoon kosher or sea salt

¼ teaspoon black pepper

8 slices baguette or slim-sized crusty whole-grain bread

2 ounces cheese (such as mozzarella, Manchego, or Monterey Jack), cut into 8 slices

French onion soup is typically made with beef broth, but Deanna wanted to perfect a meat-free version for this book (and her vegetarian mom), so she used her Veggie Scraps Broth (page 120) and added barley for extra fiber, protein, and hearty texture. And, as an added sustainability bonus, this recipe is made in a slow cooker for convenience and to save energy; caramelizing onions and cooking barley on an electric range uses much more power. While perhaps not the most authentic Mediterranean recipe, this super flavorful soup features all Mediterranean ingredient staples—except for the soy sauce, which we use to add umami (meaty flavor) to meatless dishes.

Drizzle the oil into a 6-quart slow cooker. Spread the onions over the bottom. Sprinkle the barley on top and then add the broth, wine, soy sauce, thyme, bay leaf, salt, and pepper. Cover and cook on high power for 4 hours.

About 15 minutes before you're ready to serve the soup, arrange the top oven rack about 4 inches under the broiler and preheat the broiler to high. Place the baguette slices on a large rimmed baking sheet and top each slice with a slice of cheese. Broil for 2 to 3 minutes or until the cheese is melted (watch carefully so the bread does not burn). (Alternatively, you could use your toaster oven.)

To serve, remove the bay leaf. Place a piece of cheese bread in each of eight bowls and ladle the soup on top (or ladle in the soup first and top with the cheese bread). Garnish with fresh thyme if desired.

Healthy Kitchen Hack: Make this soup a mash-up of French onion and mushroom-barley by adding mushrooms. Mushrooms are a super sustainable vegetable as they need only a small amount of space, water, and energy to produce a high yield. Add 2 to 3 cups of sliced mushrooms, such as button or cremini, with the broth to the slow cooker.

Per Serving: Calories: 282; Total Fat: 6g; Saturated Fat: 2g; Cholesterol: 6mg; Sodium: 557mg; Total Carbohydrates: 48g; Fiber: 7g; Protein: 9g

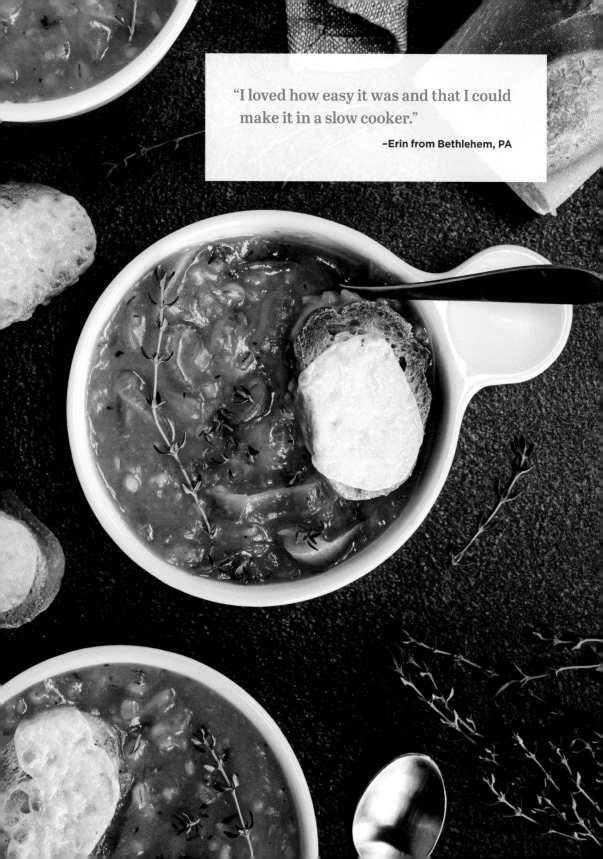

"I loved how easy it was and that I could make it in a slow cooker."

–Erin from Bethlehem, PA

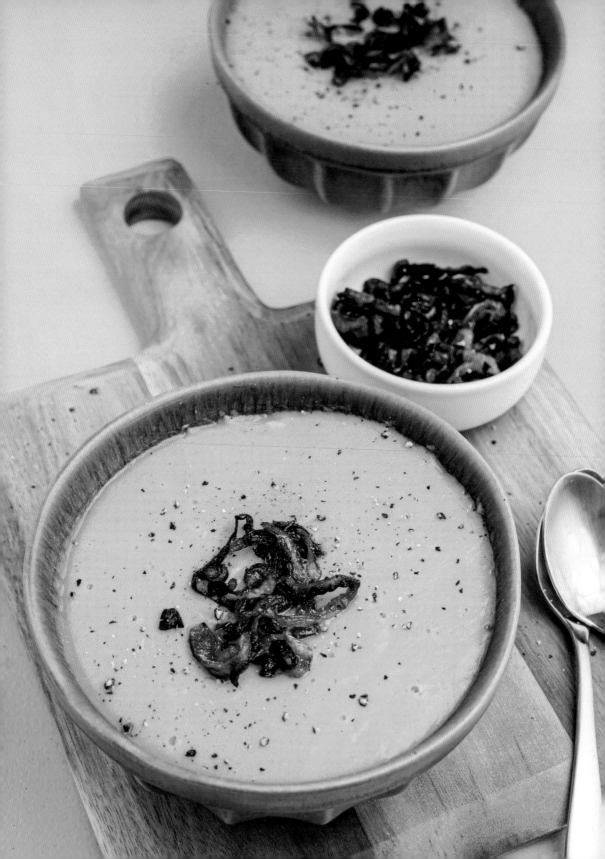

Smoky Split Pea Soup with Frizzled Onions

SERVES 6
Prep time: 10 minutes
Cook time: 40 minutes

1 lime

3 tablespoons extra-virgin olive oil, divided

8 ounces carrots (3 medium), halved lengthwise and cut into 1-inch pieces

3 garlic cloves, minced

1 tablespoon ground cumin

2 teaspoons smoked paprika

½ teaspoon kosher or sea salt

8 ounces uncooked yellow or green split peas (about 1 cup plus 2 tablespoons), rinsed

1 small onion (any type), halved and thinly sliced

½ teaspoon black pepper

Not all Serena's kids are fans of lentils, but they all love split peas—a sustainable superstar ingredient (learn more in this recipe's Healthy Kitchen Hack). So, Serena did a split pea swap in her favorite North African lentil recipe and this soup was born. If you like split pea and ham soup, you'll adore this vegetarian version (promise!), where smoked paprika and caramelized onions deliver that essential layer of smoky goodness. We like to use yellow split peas (look for them in the international aisle at your local store) because they give the soup a gorgeous golden hue, but you can also use green split peas—as long as you are good with the color being, well . . . pea-green!

Using a Microplane or citrus zester, grate the zest from the lime into a large pot or Dutch oven. (Reserve the lime for finishing the soup.) Add 2 tablespoons oil to the pot and turn the heat to medium. Add the carrots, garlic, cumin, smoked paprika, and salt and cook for about 2 minutes, stirring frequently, until the garlic just begins to turn golden and the spices are fragrant. Add the split peas and 8 cups water and bring to a boil over high heat. Cover, turn the heat down to medium, and cook for 20 minutes, stirring occasionally. Remove the lid and cook until the carrots and peas are tender, an additional 10 minutes or so. Turn off the heat.

With an immersion blender, puree the soup. (If using a regular blender, carefully puree the mixture in batches, then return it to the pot to warm before serving.)

While the soup cooks, pour the remaining 1 tablespoon oil into a large skillet over medium-high heat. Add the onion and cook, stirring frequently, until the slices turn dark golden brown or even become charred, about 10 minutes. Transfer the cooked onion to a small serving bowl.

When ready to serve, cut the lime in half and squeeze the lime juice into the soup. Add the pepper and stir

continued

to combine. Serve the frizzled onions alongside the soup to use as a topping.

Healthy Kitchen Hack: Split peas and lentils are both considered legumes, which are critical plants for regenerating the health of soil for growing other crops. Split peas are a type of green pea that is grown to be dried (compared to sweet peas that you can eat raw or cooked). Once dried, the outer skin is removed and the pea is split in half. Green split peas are a bit sweeter than the yellow variety. You can interchange them with any recipe that calls for lentils.

Per Serving: Calories: 230; Total Fat: 8g; Saturated Fat: 1g; Cholesterol: 0mg; Sodium: 208mg; Total Carbohydrates: 32g; Fiber: 12g; Protein: 10g

"This was SO delish—it was flavorful and different from typical green split pea soups. I added extra smoked paprika and cumin—will definitely make it again!"

—Karen from Blue Bell, PA

Tomato-Basil Pastina Soup with Cheese Crisps

SERVES 6
Prep time: 10 minutes
Cook time: 20 minutes

1 tablespoon extra-virgin olive oil

1 medium onion (any type), chopped

3 garlic cloves, minced

½ teaspoon smoked paprika

2 (28-ounce) cans crushed tomatoes, divided

4 cups Veggie Scraps Broth (page 120) or low-sodium vegetable broth

1 teaspoon honey

½ teaspoon black pepper, divided

¼ teaspoon kosher or sea salt

1 cup (8 ounces) uncooked pastina or acini de pepe pasta

½ cup grated Manchego or Parmesan cheese (about 2 ounces)

Pastina soup is Deanna's childhood comfort food from many meals in her grandmother's cozy rowhouse kitchen in the Italian American section of Philadelphia. Here we do a mash-up of Nana's chicken broth–based soup with a flavorful tomato soup. The recipe takes advantage of one of our favorite Mediterranean pantry staples: canned tomatoes. And our tempting cheese crisps make the perfect soup accompaniment (see the Hack for more uses), but if you want to make this soup vegan, top with our Toasted Squash Seeds (page 61) instead and replace the honey with an equal amount of sugar (but don't skip the sweetener—the small amount of sweet tames the acidity from the tomatoes).

Heat the oil in a large stockpot or Dutch oven over medium heat. Add the onion and cook, stirring frequently, for 4 minutes. Add the garlic and smoked paprika and cook, stirring frequently, for 1 minute. Pour in about 1 cup crushed tomatoes, stir, and heat for 1 minute.

Remove from the stove, ladle into a blender (or use an immersion blender in the pot), and puree until smooth. Return the tomato puree to the pot and stir in the remaining crushed tomatoes, broth, honey, ¼ teaspoon pepper, and salt. Return the pot to the stove over medium-high heat and bring to a boil. Add the pastina and lower the heat to medium; cook at a simmer for at least 15 minutes, until the pastina is done, stirring every few minutes so the pasta doesn't stick to the bottom. The longer the soup simmers, the more flavorful it will be.

While the soup simmers with the pasta, preheat the oven to 350°F and line a large rimmed baking sheet with parchment paper. Spoon the cheese into 12 portions (about 2 teaspoons each) in 2-inch circles on the sheet. Sprinkle the remaining ¼ teaspoon pepper over the cheese circles. Bake for 8 to 10 minutes, until the cheese has melted into lacy,

continued

golden-brown crisps. Remove and place the sheet on a wire rack to let the cheese crisps cool slightly.

To serve, ladle the soup into six bowls and top with two crisps per bowl.

Healthy Kitchen Hack: Just like Serena's clever method for using up the odds and ends in your cheese drawer for her Miscellaneous Toasted Cheese with Artichokes (page 129), you can make these cheese crisps with any bits of aged cheese you may have hanging out in your fridge. Try them with cheddar, Asiago, Pecorino Romano, Gruyère, and/or Gouda. Besides using them as soup toppings, toss them into green salads (crouton upgrade!), crush them over roasted veggies, or add them to our Toasted Squash Seeds and Cheese Board (page 61).

Per Serving: Calories: 291; Total Fat: 5g; Saturated Fat: 2g; Cholesterol: 5mg; Sodium: 650mg; Total Carbohydrates: 49g; Fiber: 6g; Protein: 9g

Any-Day Bouillabaisse

SERVES 6
Prep time: 5 minutes
Cook time: 15 minutes

Somewhere between a stew and a soup, this hearty Southern French seafood "st-oup" originated from Marseilles, a port city on the Mediterranean. While French families often have their own variation of it, many start with a classic base of homemade broth. It's this broth from scratch that we adapted—see this recipe's Healthy Kitchen Hack, which is one of our most referenced Hacks throughout the book! We add garlic, onions, tomatoes, and seasonings to flavor this delicious dish. And our sustainable seafood twist? Relying on canned shellfish and frozen white fish, which also makes this easy to whip up from a well-stocked pantry and freezer any day. Serve it with the traditional toasted baguette, crackers, or just about any bread (like pita, multigrain, sourdough) you have on hand to sop up the robust broth.

2 tablespoons extra-virgin olive oil

1 cup chopped onion (any type)

3 garlic cloves, divided

½ teaspoon dried thyme

¼ teaspoon ground turmeric

1 bay leaf

2 large tomatoes, diced, *or* 1 (14.5-ounce) can diced tomatoes, drained (liquid saved for another use)

2 cups Veggie Scraps Broth (recipe in the Hack) or low-sodium vegetable broth

2 (6.5-ounce) cans chopped or minced clams, drained and liquid reserved

2 (4-ounce) tins smoked mussels or smoked oysters in olive oil, drained and liquid reserved

1 (4-ounce) frozen skinless thin fish fillet (from the More Sustainable Seafood Choices list on page 19)

¼ teaspoon black pepper

1 lemon

¼ cup chopped fresh parsley, leaves and stems

8 small baguette slices *or* 4 Italian bread slices

Heat the oil in a large stockpot over medium heat. Add the onion and cook, stirring occasionally, for 4 minutes. Mince 2 garlic cloves and add them along with the thyme, turmeric, and bay leaf and cook, stirring frequently, for 30 seconds. Add the tomatoes and cook, stirring frequently, for 1 minute. Add the broth and liquid from the clams and mussels (but not the seafood itself yet) and bring to a boil, then turn the heat down to medium-low and add the fish fillet. Cook for 5 minutes, then add the clams, mussels, and pepper. Stir and cook until warmed through, 1 to 2 minutes. Remove from the heat and break up the fish with a fork in the pot. Using a Microplane or citrus zester, grate the zest from the lemon over the pot. Cut the lemon into wedges and set aside. Mix the fresh parsley into the pot. Remove the bay leaf.

continued

About 15 minutes before you're ready to serve the soup, arrange the top oven rack about 4 inches under the broiler and preheat the broiler to high. Place the baguette slices on a rimmed baking sheet and broil for 1 minute, flip the slices, and broil for an additional 1 to 2 minutes (watch carefully to prevent burning). (Alternatively, you could use your toaster oven.) Cut the remaining garlic clove in half and rub one side on each piece of toast (save the remaining garlic for another recipe).

Serve the soup with the toasted bread slices and lemon wedges.

Healthy Kitchen Hack: Throughout this book, we've encouraged you to throw your veggie scraps into a freezer container to make an easy Veggie Scraps Broth. Here's how: In a large stockpot, combine 4 cups veggie scraps (like carrot peels, broccoli stems, onion skins, tough ends of celery and asparagus, etc.), 6 sprigs thyme or rosemary (or 2 teaspoons dried), a handful of fresh parsley or cilantro, 2 bay leaves, and about 12 black peppercorns (or you can season with ground black pepper to taste when the broth is finished). Pour in 8 cups water (or a combination of water and the saved liquid brine from canned/jarred veggies like tomatoes, olives, and artichokes) and bring to a boil over medium-high heat. Partially cover, reduce the heat to medium-low, and simmer for 45 minutes. Strain out the solids (if you're able, compost them!). Cool the broth for about 20 minutes, then store in jars in the refrigerator for up to 5 days or in 2- to 4-cup portions in freezer-safe containers in the freezer for up to 6 months. Makes approximately 8 cups.

Per Serving: Calories: 412; Total Fat: 14g; Saturated Fat: 2g; Cholesterol: 139mg; Sodium: 789mg; Total Carbohydrates: 40g; Fiber: 5g; Protein: 28g

Cheesy Broccoli and Greens Soup with Za'atar

SERVES 6
Prep time: 15 minutes
Cook time: 30 minutes

4 cups chopped raw broccoli (about 2 large broccoli heads with peeled stalks) *or* 2½ cups chopped cooked broccoli

2–3 tablespoons extra-virgin olive oil, divided

½ teaspoon black pepper, divided

¼ teaspoon kosher or sea salt, divided

8 cups dark leafy greens of choice (about 2 large bunches; see headnote), washed

2 garlic cloves, minced

1½ teaspoons za'atar, divided

4 cups Veggie Scraps Broth (page 120), low-sodium vegetable broth, or water

1 cup 2% milk

½ cup grated Parmesan cheese

¼ cup plain 2% Greek yogurt

When colder weather arrives for the long haul, Deanna adds this wholesome recipe—a Middle Eastern twist on the classic broccoli cheese soup—to her weekly meal rotation. It's a smart "use up those dark leafies" strategy and also a deceptively delish way to serve up spinach, kale, chard, mustard greens, and/or collards to family members who might not usually be so eager to eat them. If you don't have za'atar on hand (though we highly recommend adding it to your spice drawer), swap in dried thyme, smoked paprika, or ground cumin for that extra layer of Mediterranean flavor.

If you're starting with raw broccoli, preheat the oven to 450°F. Coat a large rimmed baking sheet with cooking spray.

In a large bowl, toss the broccoli with 1 tablespoon oil, ¼ teaspoon pepper, and ⅛ teaspoon salt. Spread out the raw broccoli on the prepared baking sheet. Roast for 10 minutes or until the broccoli starts to darken, stirring once halfway through.

Wash the dark leafy greens and remove the stems. Finely chop the stems, then coarsely chop the leaves. Set aside separately.

Heat 1 tablespoon oil in a large pot or Dutch oven over medium heat. Add the garlic and 1 teaspoon za'atar and cook for 1 minute, stirring frequently. Add the chopped greens stems and cook for 2 minutes. Then add about half of the chopped leaves, cook for about 1 minute until they wilt down a bit, and then add the remaining leaves. Cook, stirring occasionally, until the greens are completely wilted; this will take an additional 2 to 4 minutes depending on how hearty your greens are.

Stir in the cooked broccoli, vegetable broth, milk, remaining ¼ teaspoon pepper, and remaining ⅛ teaspoon salt. Cook for about 15 minutes or until the broccoli and greens are completely soft.

continued

Cheesy Broccoli and Greens Soup with Za'atar *(continued)*

With an immersion blender, puree the soup until completely smooth. (If using a regular blender or food processor, carefully puree the mixture in batches, then return it to the pot.) Stir in the cheese and reduce to low heat. Cook until the cheese melts, stirring occasionally, 1 to 2 minutes.

For the soup topping, in a small bowl, whisk together the yogurt, remaining 1 tablespoon oil, and remaining ½ teaspoon za'atar. Ladle the soup into bowls and top each with a dollop of the savory yogurt. Any leftover soup will keep in an airtight container for about 5 days in the refrigerator or for several months in the freezer.

Healthy Kitchen Hack: When buying fresh broccoli, select the entire head (not just the crowns!) because the stalks are actually the sweetest part of the plant. Before chopping, peel the tough skin off the stalk to get to the tender inner part (and save to your Veggie Scraps freezer bag to make the Veggie Scraps Broth on page 120).

Per Serving (with 2 teaspoons yogurt topping): Calories: 165; Total Fat: 11g; Saturated Fat: 3g; Cholesterol: 11mg; Sodium: 339mg; Total Carbohydrates: 12g; Fiber: 3g; Protein: 7g

"I was surprised that so many of my kids and grandkids actually liked this soup! I really hadn't heard about za'atar before this recipe, but we liked it and will use it more often. The yogurt soup topping was delicious."

—Judy from Edwardsville, IL

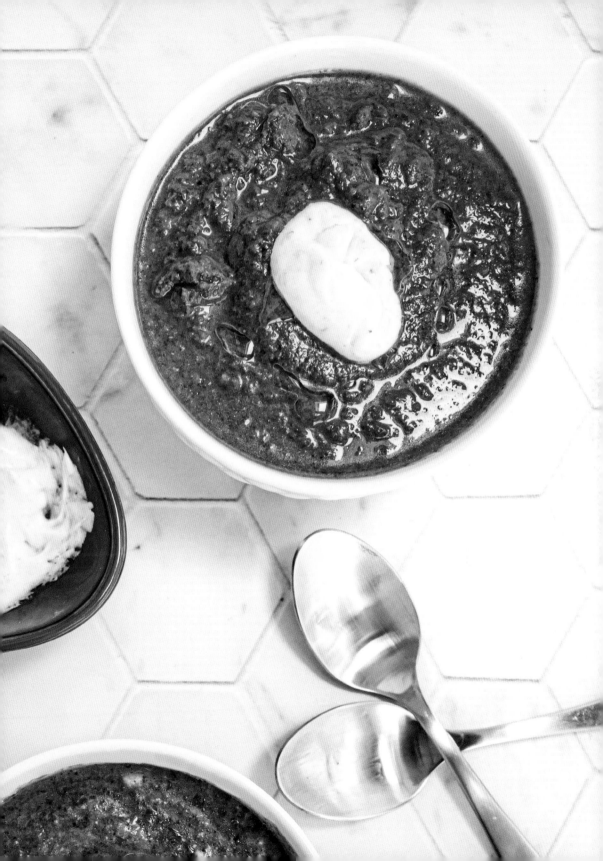

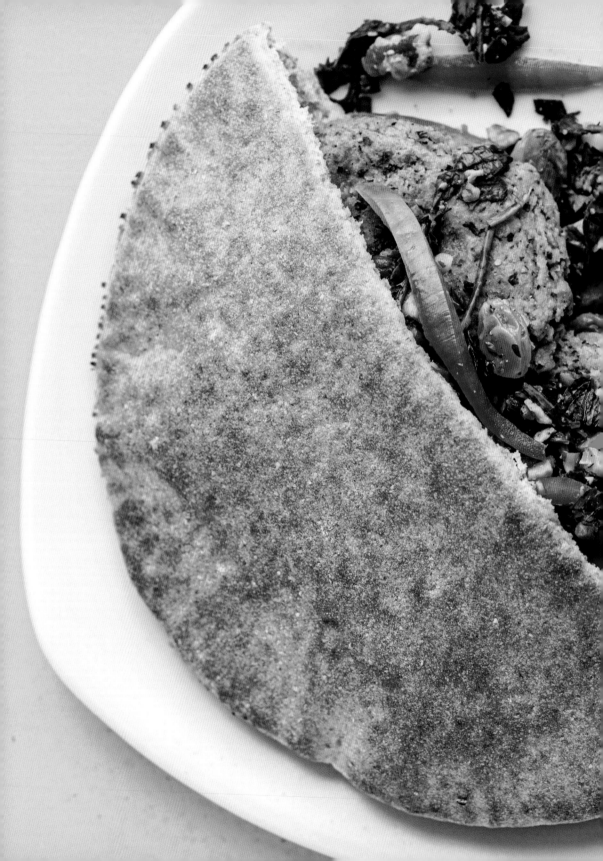

Sandwiches and Pizza

Hummus and Za'atar Chicken Salad Sandwiches

SERVES 6
Prep time: 15 minutes

1 orange

1 (15-ounce) can chickpeas, drained and liquid reserved

2 tablespoons extra-virgin olive oil

2 tablespoons tahini or peanut butter

2 teaspoons za'atar, divided

3 cups shredded or cubed cooked chicken (from about 1½ pounds cooked bone-in chicken pieces; see Hack)

4 celery stalks and leaves, diced (about 1 cup)

1 (2.25-ounce) can sliced black olives, drained (liquid saved for another use), *or* ½ cup sliced green olives

2 scallions (green onions), green and white parts, thinly sliced
Save the stem roots!
See page 70

¼ teaspoon kosher or sea salt

¼ teaspoon black pepper

1½ teaspoons red wine vinegar or apple cider vinegar

4 whole-grain sandwich rolls

Lettuce, for serving (optional)

Ditch the mayo and embrace the hummus when it comes to your next chicken salad sandwich! Besides being a yummy way to use up leftover cooked chicken, this protein-packed (30 grams per serving!) meal is equally delicious on rolls or in pita or served on a bed of greens. This delicious hummus is flavored with orange plus some za'atar spice, though you could also try the recipe with ¾ cup of our Pumpkin Hummus (page 63) or your favorite store-bought hummus; make the chicken salad ahead and refrigerate it overnight to maximize all these flavors. Sometimes Deanna will switch the olives for chopped figs, apricots, or golden raisins for a hit of sweetness.

Using a Microplane or citrus zester, grate the zest from the orange over a food processor or blender. Cut the orange in half and squeeze in 2 tablespoons juice (reserve the remaining juice for the chicken salad). Add the chickpeas, 3 tablespoons of the reserved chickpea liquid, oil, tahini, and 1 teaspoon za'atar. Process until smooth, adding another tablespoon or two reserved chickpea liquid until the hummus reaches a mayonnaise-like consistency. Set aside.

In a large mixing bowl, mix together the chicken, celery, olives, scallions, remaining orange juice, remaining 1 teaspoon za'atar, salt, and pepper until all the chicken is moistened. Add ¾ cup of the hummus (save the remaining for our Toasted Seeds and Cheese Plate on page 61, Spicy Fish Shawarma Bowls on page 225, or Parsley, Pistachio, and Bulgur Beef Koftas on page 240). Gently stir, then add the vinegar and mix until all the ingredients are just incorporated. Serve on rolls with lettuce if desired, or chill in an airtight container in the refrigerator overnight for flavors to meld and use within 4 days.

Note: Peanut butter may be substituted for tahini, but the recipe will no longer be nut-free.

Healthy Kitchen Hack: Here's our easy poached chicken method with the bonus of homemade chicken broth! Put 1 to 2 pounds of bone-in chicken breasts and/or thighs in a large stockpot. Cover with water by 1 inch. Add any or all of the following "tired" looking veggies: a carrot (cut in half), celery stalk (cut in half), onion (cut in quarters), 2 or 3 smashed garlic cloves and 3 or 4 sprigs rosemary or thyme. Cover and bring to a boil. Reduce the heat to low and cook for about 15 minutes (still covered) or until the chicken's internal temperature reaches 165°F on a meat thermometer. Remove the chicken, cool slightly, and then use in a recipe or refrigerate. Strain the broth (compost the veggies!) and store in a jar in the refrigerator for up to 7 days or in a freezer-safe container in the freezer for up to 6 months.

Per Serving: Calories: 383; Total Fat: 12g; Saturated Fat: 2g; Cholesterol: 83mg; Sodium: 648mg; Total Carbohydrates: 33g; Fiber: 5g; Protein: 30g

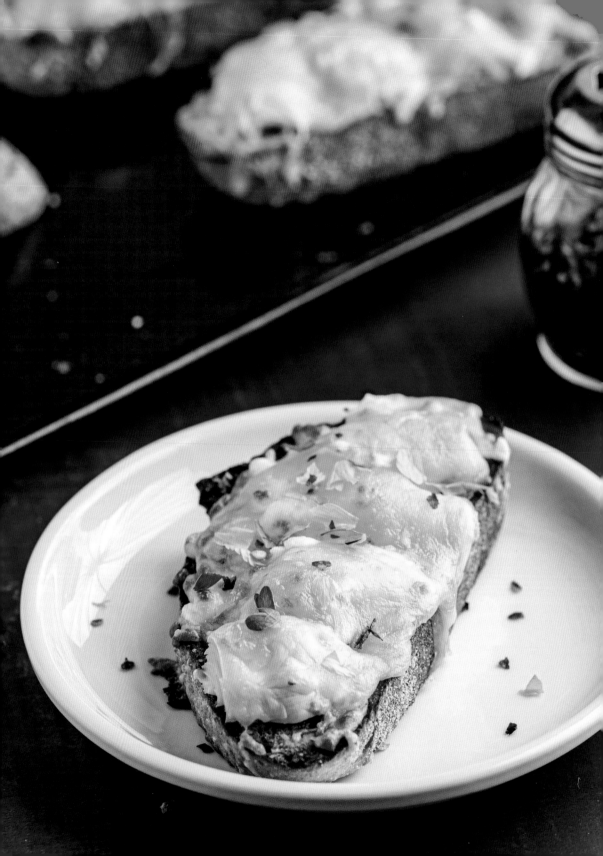

Miscellaneous Toasted Cheese with Artichokes

SERVES 4
Prep time: 10 minutes
Cook time: 5 minutes

4 ounces shredded cheeses (about 1½ cups; see headnote)

1 tablespoon extra-virgin olive oil

4 slices whole-grain crusty bread or any leftover bread (see note)

1 garlic clove, cut in half

⅓ cup chopped celery leaves *or* chopped fresh parsley, cilantro, or basil

1 (14-ounce) can quartered artichoke hearts (not marinated), drained (liquid saved for another use) and patted dry

¼ teaspoon black pepper

⅛ teaspoon crushed red pepper (optional)

This toasted sandwich is your ooey-gooey, comfort food way to use up those dibs and dabs of cheese in the fridge. Preferably, use a mix of harder cheeses (such as Parmesan and/or cheddar), semi-soft (like mozzarella), and softer cheeses (such as feta, goat, and/or cream cheese) to hold the spread together—but any cheeses you have will do! In France, this solution to the leftover cheese challenge is called fromage fort. Serena's grandmother called it "cheese spread" and smeared it on celery sticks to serve alongside canned tomato soup for lunch. Inspired by Grandma Evelyn, we added a few celery leaf sprigs to our version of this open-faced grilled cheese to balance out its rich, melty decadence—and because celery leaves often get tossed! And for a Mediterranean spin, we add artichokes (one of our favorite canned goods staples) for a tasty texture contrast while providing a good dose of healthy prebiotic fiber.

Arrange the top oven rack about 4 inches from the broiler. Preheat the broiler to high.

In a medium bowl, using a fork, stir and mash the cheeses with the oil until a somewhat cohesive spread forms; if the spread doesn't come together, add a bit more soft cheese or olive oil.

Place the bread slices on a rimmed baking sheet and broil until just barely toasted on one side, 1 to 2 minutes. Rub the toasted sides of the bread with a garlic half (save the cut garlic halves for another recipe). Lay the celery leaves over the bread, leaving a ½-inch border. Top each sandwich with 4 or 5 artichoke quarters (save the remaining artichokes for another use). Using a silicone spatula and/or your fingers, sprinkle and press the cheese spread over the artichokes and celery leaves, pressing all the way to the edges (to prevent the edges from burning). Sprinkle each piece with the black pepper.

Broil until the cheese is bubbling and just beginning to turn golden brown, 2 to 3 minutes; watch carefully so

continued

the bread doesn't burn. Sprinkle with crushed red pepper if desired and serve.

Note: If you're using a baguette-style bread, slice it in half lengthwise and then cut into serving pieces.

Healthy Kitchen Hack: Around the world, this cheese spread is made in a variety of ways using leftover cheese typically moistened with wine, beer, or butter; in Mediterranean style, we use olive oil. To get a more uniform consistency, especially if you are using up hard aged cheese, you can whizz it in your food processor. Get creative and mix in leftover herbs, sun-dried tomatoes, dried fruits, and/or chopped olives. Besides toasted on bread, enjoy this cheese spread on crackers, pizza, raw veggie sticks, or fruit slices. Mix it into warm pasta or whole grains; or serve in a small bowl on our Toasted Squash Seeds and Cheese Board (page 61).

Per Serving: Calories: 234; **Total Fat:** 11g; **Saturated Fat:** 5g; **Cholesterol:** 26mg; **Sodium:** 468mg; **Total Carbohydrates:** 22g; **Fiber:** 5g; **Protein:** 10g

Spanish Broccoli-Stuffed Calzones Two Ways

SERVES 8
Prep time: 20 minutes
Cook time: 25 minutes

Classic Italian "pizza pockets" get a Spanish-inspired stuffing in this dish, which features three of our staple recipes: Speedy Pizza Dough (page 138), Romesco Sauce (page 91), and Made-in-Minutes Homemade Ricotta Cheese (page 48). Here, we nudge broccoli lovers to expand their flavor horizons with two different stuffing options—that are, in fact, pretty yummy served on their own or tossed with hot pasta for days you want to skip the dough (though we do encourage you to try these calzones at least once). And if you aren't feeling ambitious, or didn't make all those staple recipes ahead of time, grab some refrigerated pizza dough, jarred or canned pizza sauce, and/or store-bought ricotta—it's all good!

5 cups finely chopped raw broccoli (about 2 large heads with peeled stalks; see Hack) *or* 1 (1-pound) bag frozen chopped broccoli, thawed and drained

2 tablespoons extra-virgin olive oil

2 garlic cloves, minced

1 teaspoon honey

¼ teaspoon kosher or sea salt

1 batch Speedy Pizza Dough (page 138) *or* 1½ pounds refrigerated or thawed frozen pizza dough, at room temperature

Choose one of the following fillings:

ROMESCO CHEESE FILLING

½ batch Romesco Sauce (page 91) *or* 1½ cups your favorite pizza sauce

¾ cup grated Parmesan or Pecorino Romano cheese

RICOTTA CHEESE FILLING

2 batches Made-in-Minutes Homemade Ricotta Cheese recipe (page 48) *or* 1½ cups store-bought part-skim ricotta cheese

¾ cup grated Parmesan or Pecorino Romano cheese

1 large egg, lightly whisked

¼ teaspoon smoked paprika

¼ teaspoon kosher or sea salt

¼ teaspoon black pepper

Arrange the oven racks to the upper-middle and lower-middle positions. Place a large rimmed baking sheet on the lower-middle rack, then preheat the oven to 450°F (with the sheet inside).

In a large bowl, toss the broccoli, oil, garlic, honey, and salt with your hands or tongs until the broccoli is fully coated. Carefully remove the preheated baking sheet from the oven and spread the broccoli onto the hot baking sheet. Bake for 5 minutes

continued

or until the broccoli is fork-tender and just starts to brown, remove from the oven, and scrape back into the same large bowl.

While the broccoli bakes, prepare the dough. Lightly flour your work surface and divide the dough into eight equal portions. Roll each portion into an 8-inch circle.

Add your choice of filling ingredients to the bowl with the warm broccoli and mix well.

Wipe off the broccoli baking sheet and coat it and another large rimmed baking sheet with cooking spray. Spoon some filling onto one half of a dough circle, leaving a ½-inch border. Fold the dough over to cover the filling, pinching to seal around the edges (the calzone will be in a half moon shape). Press down on the seal firmly with a fork or your fingers to make sure the calzone is fully sealed. Carefully transfer the calzone to one of the prepared baking sheets. Repeat to form the remaining calzones.

Bake for 10 minutes, then quickly switch the top baking sheet to the bottom rack and vice versa so the calzones bake evenly. Bake for another 7 to 8 minutes or until the tops and edges just start to turn golden brown. Remove from the oven and cool for about 5 minutes before serving.

Healthy Kitchen Hack: These calzones freeze well. Simply bake according to the recipe directions and let them cool completely. Then, wrap them individually in foil and store in the freezer for up to 3 months. To reheat one, unwrap and warm in a toaster oven at 350°F for about 20 minutes. Or heat in a skillet over medium heat for 3 minutes, covered. Flip and heat for 3 more minutes. If the filling is still cool, turn heat to medium-low (to prevent burning the crust), and heat for a few more minutes. To speed up the warming process, first thaw the calzone in the refrigerator a few hours before reheating.

Per Serving (with romesco filling): Calories: 346; Total Fat: 11g; Saturated Fat: 4g; Cholesterol: 15mg; Sodium: 598mg; Total Carbohydrates: 47g; Fiber: 5g; Protein: 18g
Per Serving (with ricotta filling): Calories: 367; Total Fat: 12g; Saturated Fat: 5g; Cholesterol: 50mg; Sodium: 573mg; Total Carbohydrates: 46g; Fiber: 5g; Protein: 21g

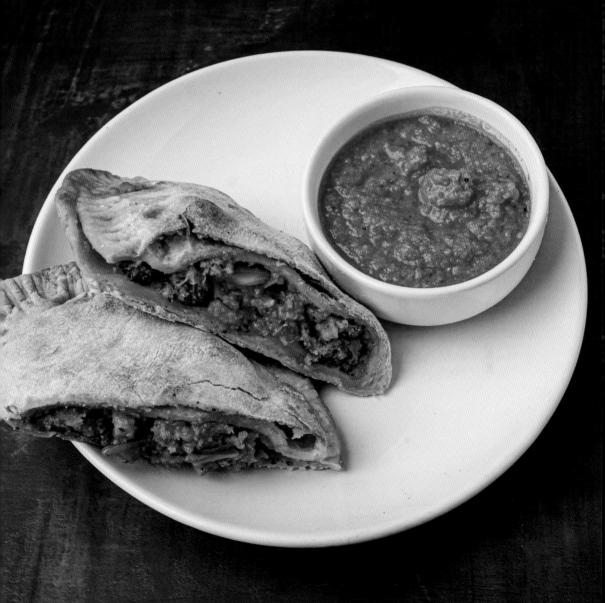

Falafel with Pickled Onion Herb Relish

SERVES 4
Prep time: 20 minutes
Cook time: 15 minutes

⅓ cup white wine vinegar or rice vinegar

1 tablespoon sugar

¾ teaspoon kosher or sea salt, divided

1 cup thinly sliced red onion

¼ teaspoon crushed red pepper

1 (15-ounce) can chickpeas, drained (liquid saved for another use) and rinsed

2 cups chopped fresh parsley, cilantro, or basil, leaves and stems, divided

3 tablespoons quick or old-fashioned rolled oats

2 garlic cloves, chopped

1 tablespoon ground cumin

½ teaspoon baking powder

¼ teaspoon black pepper

3 tablespoons extra-virgin olive oil, divided

¼ cup golden or regular raisins

¼ cup chopped walnuts

2 whole-wheat pita breads, halved and toasted

In each of our cookbooks, there's always one recipe that we tested and tinkered with an endless number of times (or so it seems) to get just right. Luckily, even the early renditions of these crunchy cumin-scented chickpea sandwiches with a tangy herb and onion spread were so delicious that Serena's family didn't mind eating them many, many nights in a row. Getting the texture just right proved to be the tricky part, and in the end, pan-frying won out for the crispiest golden fritters. Make these yourself to see why falafel is such a popular staple street food throughout the Mediterranean!

Put a large plate in your freezer to use later for forming the falafel patties.

First, make the pickled onions. In a medium bowl, stir together the vinegar, sugar, and ½ teaspoon salt until dissolved. Mix in the onion and crushed red pepper. Let sit for at least 10 minutes while you make the falafel.

In a food processor or high-powered blender, start to pulse the chickpeas, 1 cup parsley, oats, garlic, cumin, baking powder, remaining ¼ teaspoon salt, and black pepper while slowly drizzling in 1 tablespoon oil (or you can use a fork instead to mash all the ingredients together in a bowl). Continue to pulse until all the ingredients are combined and the mixture sticks together with only a few smaller chunks of chickpeas remaining.

Remove the plate from the freezer and coat with cooking spray. Scoop the chickpea mixture into 8 even portions on the plate. Flatten each portion with your hand to about 2 inches in diameter and ½ inch thick; press around the edges so the falafel patties are tightly packed to help prevent them from falling apart when cooking. Return the plate with the falafel to the freezer for 5 minutes.

While the plate chills, heat 1 tablespoon oil in a large skillet over medium heat. Line a large plate with a clean towel. Remove the plate from the freezer and add 4 falafel patties to the skillet. Cook until golden, 5 to 6 minutes, flipping halfway through. Transfer to the towel-lined plate and cover to keep warm while cooking the remaining 4 falafel patties in the remaining 1 tablespoon oil.

To the bowl with the pickled onion, add the remaining 1 cup parsley, raisins, and walnuts and stir to combine.

Fill each pita bread with 2 falafel patties, top with the pickled onion relish, and serve immediately.

Healthy Kitchen Hack: While we think the pickled onion herb relish takes this sandwich to the next level, you can certainly top your falafel patties with other condiments or ingredients you already have in your fridge or pantry instead, such as capers, olives, roasted red peppers, sun-dried tomatoes, hot sauce, or even the humble but tried-and-true dill pickle.

Per Serving: Calories: 342; **Total Fat:** 18g; **Saturated Fat:** 2g; **Cholesterol:** 0mg; **Sodium:** 540mg; **Total Carbohydrates:** 40g; **Fiber:** 9g; **Protein:** 9g

"The pickled onion herb topping made the sandwich really flavorful—and the whole thing was so colorful with purple onions and green herbs, which I loved."

—Audrey from Glen Carbon, IL

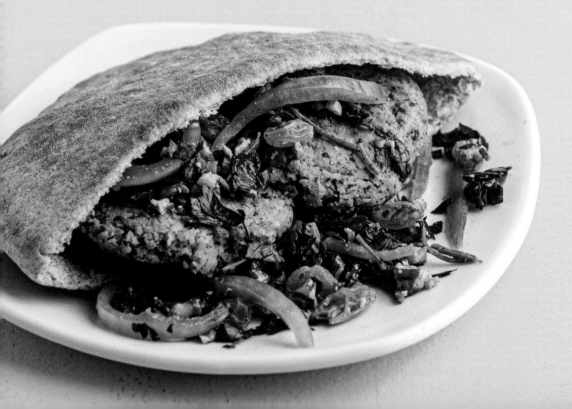

Crispy Baked Lavash Wraps with Fish and Olive Tapenade

SERVES 4
Prep time: 10 minutes
Cook time: 15 minutes

24 pitted jarred or canned olives, finely chopped

¼ cup chopped fresh parsley, leaves and stems

1 garlic clove, minced

2 lemons

1 tablespoon plus 2 teaspoons extra-virgin olive oil, divided

4 (4-ounce) frozen skinless fish fillets (from the More Sustainable Seafood Choices list on page 19), thawed

¼ teaspoon kosher or sea salt

¼ teaspoon black pepper

4 (12 × 9-inch) pieces lavash flatbread

The first time Serena tried this method of baking fish in lavash—a thin leavened Middle Eastern flatbread—the result was a bit of a revelation (making this one of her favorite recipes in the entire cookbook)! Outside the lavash becomes flaky and crispy, while inside the fish cooks up perfectly moist and tender, all paired with the vibrant flavors from the olive and herb relish spread. When shopping, look for the thin rectangular lavash in your store's bread aisle to ensure crunchy sandwich results instead of a round flatbread, which bakes up with a chewy texture.

Preheat the oven to 400°F. Spread a sheet of parchment paper on a large rimmed baking sheet.

Combine the olives, parsley, and garlic in a medium bowl. Using a Microplane or citrus zester, grate the zest from 1 lemon into the bowl, then cut the lemon in half and squeeze in the juice. Cut the other lemon in wedges for serving; set aside. Add 1 teaspoon oil to the bowl and mix to combine. Set aside.

Pat the fillets dry and sprinkle both sides with the salt and pepper. Brush one piece of lavash bread with 1 teaspoon oil. Place one piece of fish on the shorter side of the lavash, about 2 inches from the edge; spread with one-fourth of the tapenade. Fold in both long sides, then fold up the bottom and roll up the lavash; transfer to the prepared baking sheet, seam-side down. Repeat with remaining pieces of lavash, fish, and tapenade, leaving as much room as possible between the wraps on the baking sheet.

Bake until the lavash is crisp and the fish is cooked through, about 20 minutes. To test doneness, cut one wrap in half to see if the fish is opaque.

Cut each wrap in half and serve with the lemon wedges.

Healthy Kitchen Hack: People around the Mediterranean Sea eat nutrient-packed olives daily. We often rely on canned olives (typically ones that are grown in California versus being imported), and while these are usually pitted, here's a quick trick to remove pits if you buy other varieties: gently smash a few olives at a time using a coffee mug or a glass measuring cup. Then simply remove the pits from the broken pieces of olives.

Per Serving: Calories: 280; Total Fat: 11g; Saturated Fat: 1g; Cholesterol: 52mg; Sodium: 967mg; Total Carbohydrates: 19g; Fiber: 5g; Protein: 32g

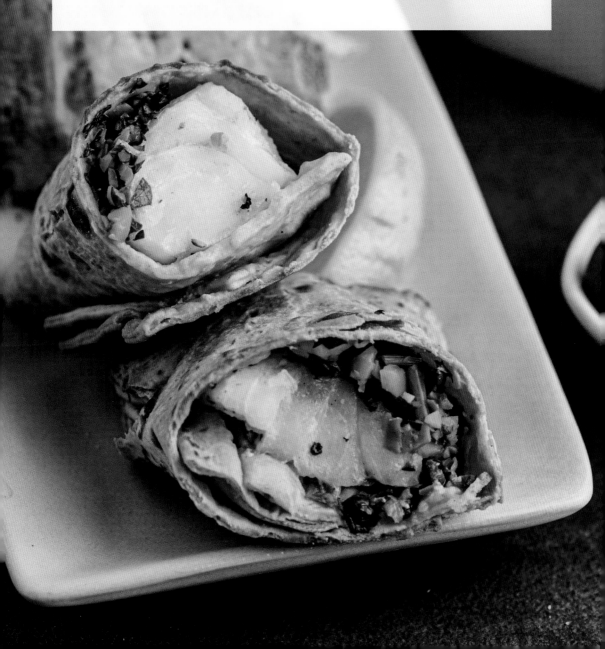

Speedy Pizza Dough

SERVES 8
Prep time: 20 minutes

2 cups all-purpose flour, plus more for kneading

1 cup whole-wheat pastry flour or white whole-wheat flour (see Hack)

1 tablespoon baking powder

¾ teaspoon kosher or sea salt

2 cups plain 2% Greek yogurt

Save gas and transportation miles by skipping the pizza pickup or delivery and make your own dough in minutes! It's so convenient that we make this no-yeast, no-rise-time recipe almost weekly. The combination of the baking powder and the acid from the yogurt rises the dough into an appealing, chewy crust. It's used in our Spanish Broccoli-Stuffed Calzones (page 131), Four Seasons Pizza Pies (page 140), and Rustic Roasted Vegetable Crostata (page 183). Bonus: this dough packs a protein punch at 11 grams per serving—and that's before you add any toppings!

In a large bowl or stand mixer bowl, measure the flours, baking powder, and salt. With a wooden spoon or spatula if mixing by hand or the dough hook attachment if using a stand mixer, mix the dry ingredients and then gradually add the yogurt, ½ cup at a time. Continue to mix until a dough begins to form. If the dough is too dry, add 1 or 2 tablespoons water (this will depend on the type of flour used).

Knead the dough on a lightly flour-dusted work surface for 1 to 2 minutes, until smooth (if the dough is too sticky when kneading, add a few teaspoons of flour to the work surface and work it in). Form the dough into a ball, cover with a dish towel, and let rest for at least 10 minutes before using. For baking directions, see the recipe for Four Seasons Pizza Pies (page 140).

Note: The recipe makes about 1½ pounds of dough and can be used to make two large pizzas or eight individual pizzas. If not using right away, store the dough after resting in a freezer-safe container in your freezer for up to 6 months. Defrost by letting the dough sit on the counter for a few hours until completely thawed.

Healthy Kitchen Hack: We've experimented with many types of whole-wheat flour over the years since they serve up more fiber and nutrients in recipes. Serena prefers white whole-wheat and Deanna's go-to is whole-wheat pastry flour, but depending on your local store, you may not have these options. Instead, you can make

"The dough is absolutely wonderful! It's so easy to prepare and work with and it's really tasty, too."

—Jessica from Silver Spring, MD

this recipe with 3 cups all-purpose flour, bread flour, or even gluten-free flour. If you keep any type of whole-wheat flour in your kitchen, store it in the freezer for the maximum shelf life (up to a year) as the bran and germ contain oils that can oxidize and cause rancidity.

Per Serving (using whole-wheat pastry flour): Calories: 206; Total Fat: 2g; Saturated Fat: 1g; Cholesterol: 6mg; Sodium: 201mg; Total Carbohydrates: 37g; Fiber: 3g; Protein: 11g

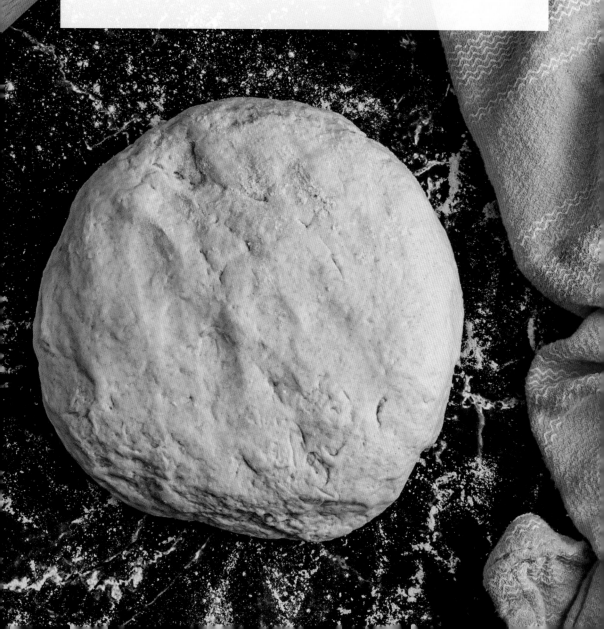

Four Seasons Pizza Pies

SERVES 8
Prep time: 10 minutes
Cook time: 15 minutes

1 batch Speedy Pizza Dough (page 138) or 1½ pounds store-bought pizza dough, at room temperature

2 teaspoons extra-virgin olive oil

6 ounces sliced or shredded mozzarella cheese (about 1½ cups)

1 (14-ounce) can quartered artichoke hearts (not marinated), drained (liquid saved for another use)

1 (14-ounce) can mushrooms pieces and stems, drained (liquid saved for another use)

1 (12-ounce) jar roasted red peppers, drained (liquid saved for another use) and thinly sliced

½ teaspoon dried oregano

2 tablespoons grated Parmesan cheese

¼ teaspoon black pepper

¼ teaspoon crushed red pepper (optional)

Inspired by a sauceless pie from one of Deanna's favorite Italian American markets, this pizza is topped with our favorite veggie pantry staples so you can make it in any season! Because we use our yogurt-based Speedy Pizza Dough (page 138), each serving provides close to 20 grams of protein, but you can also boost your seafood intake by adding some canned smoked mussels or clams to your topping mix.

Arrange the oven racks to the upper-middle and lower-middle positions. Preheat the oven to 475°F. Coat two large baking sheets with cooking spray.

Lightly flour your work surface and divide the dough into two equal portions. Roll each portion into a 13-inch circle and place on the prepared sheets. Brush each pizza crust with 1 teaspoon oil. Scatter the mozzarella over both pizzas. Top with the artichokes, mushrooms, and roasted red peppers.

Crush the dried oregano between your fingers and sprinkle over the pizzas. Top with the grated Parmesan, black pepper, and crushed red pepper if desired.

Bake for 15 to 18 minutes or until the bottom and sides of the crust start to turn golden brown. Remove from the oven, cut each pizza into 8 slices, and serve immediately.

Healthy Kitchen Hack: Grill your summer pizza pies (or any season if you're a dedicated year-round griller)! Have the dough rolled out and toppings ready to go, then heat the grill to high and brush the grates with olive oil. Coat two baking sheets with cooking spray. Place the rolled-out pizzas (without toppings) on the grill grates, cover, and grill for 2 to 3 minutes or until the bottoms are lightly charred. Using tongs, transfer the pizzas, grilled-side up, to the prepared baking sheets. Layer the toppings, then carefully slide the pizzas back onto the grill. Cook for an additional 2 to 3 minutes or until the crust is done to your liking.

Per Serving (2 slices): Calories: 321; Total Fat: 7g; Saturated Fat: 3g; Cholesterol: 20mg; Sodium: 675mg; Total Carbohydrates: 48g; Fiber: 6g; Protein: 18g

Cheesy Crab Panini

SERVES 4
Prep time: 10 minutes
Cook time: 10 minutes

1 lemon

⅓ cup plain whole-milk Greek yogurt

1 tablespoon extra-virgin olive oil

½ teaspoon Worcestershire sauce (optional)

½ teaspoon black pepper

¼ teaspoon crushed red pepper

2 (6-ounce) cans crabmeat, drained

2 scallions (green onions), green and white parts, thinly sliced
Save the stem roots! See page 70

½ cup chopped fresh basil, cilantro, or parsley, leaves and stems

1 cup shredded part-skim mozzarella cheese

1 (12-inch) whole-grain Italian loaf, cut into 4 equal sections

Made with sustainable canned crab, this pressed cheese sandwich delivers a happy contrast of flavors and textures with every bite. Sweet crabmeat and salty cheese is stuffed between crispy griddled bread, with a yogurt–olive oil spread we call "Mediterranean mayo." Serve these with a side of soup or a crisp salad for a complete meal and a taste of the ocean, even if you live far from the seashore.

Using a Microplane or citrus zester, grate the zest from the lemon over a large bowl, then cut the lemon in half and squeeze in 1 tablespoon juice. (Save the remaining lemon juice for another use.) Add the yogurt, oil, Worcestershire sauce (if using), black pepper, and crushed red pepper and whisk to combine completely.

In a colander, using a silicone spatula, press as much water out of the crabmeat as possible. Add the crabmeat to the yogurt mixture along with the scallions, basil, and cheese and mix gently to combine.

Coat a grill pan, large skillet, or panini maker with cooking spray and heat over medium-high heat.

Cut open each section of bread lengthwise without slicing all the way through. If some of the liquid has separated from the crabmeat mixture, stir it back in, then divide it equally among the bread sections. Close the sandwiches and arrange two on the heated grill pan, skillet, or panini press. If using a grill pan or skillet, put another skillet or other clean, heavy object on top of the sandwiches and grill for about 3 minutes. Flip and grill for an additional 2 to 3 minutes. If using a panini press, close and grill until the crust is golden and the cheese has melted, 3 to 5 minutes. Repeat with the other 2 sandwiches, and serve.

Healthy Kitchen Hack: Take advantage of all the canned seafood aisle has to offer to make different and unique types of panini. Canned tuna works great (think tuna melt), as do canned salmon, smoked trout, and even sardines.

Per Serving: Calories: 265; Total Fat: 10g; Saturated Fat: 4g; Cholesterol: 52mg; Sodium: 665mg; Total Carbohydrates: 29g; Fiber: 6g; Protein: 19g

DAIRY-FREE, EGG-FREE, VEGAN

Turkish Tomato Flatbreads (Lahmacun)

SERVES 4
Prep time: 5 minutes
Cook time: 40 minutes

½ cup walnuts

4 (7- to 8-inch) whole-wheat pita breads

3 tablespoons extra-virgin olive oil, divided

1 medium onion (any type), diced

1 red bell pepper, seeded and chopped

1 green bell pepper, seeded and chopped

1 tablespoon ground cumin

1 teaspoon sweet paprika (optional)

½ teaspoon black pepper

¼ teaspoon kosher or sea salt

¼ teaspoon smoked paprika *or* ⅛ teaspoon crushed red pepper

3 tablespoons tomato paste

2 tablespoons red wine vinegar

1 cup chopped fresh parsley or cilantro, leaves and stems

These pizza-like, cheeseless flatbreads are popular in Turkey, Lebanon, Syria, and other Middle Eastern regions. Every cook has their own favorite way of making lahmacun, but the classic sauce ingredients usually include tomatoes, onions, sweet peppers, cumin, and fiery chile peppers. The sauce is cooked down with ground lamb, spread onto the dough, and then topped with lots of fresh parsley. Our vegetarian version substitutes crushed walnuts for the meat and uses one of our favorite techniques for adding an extra oomph of rich flavor: caramelized tomato paste.

Preheat the oven to 375°F. Coat two large rimmed baking sheets with cooking spray.

In a reusable food bag or resealable plastic bag, crush the walnuts into very small crumbles using a rolling pin or heavy skillet. Set aside.

Using kitchen shears or a knife, slit each pita around the edges, open, and pull apart so you have 8 rounds. Place the rounds, cut-side down, on the prepared baking sheets. Set aside.

Heat 2 tablespoons oil in a large skillet over medium heat. Add the onion and cook, stirring occasionally, for 5 minutes, until they begin to soften. Add the bell peppers and cook, stirring occasionally, until they begin to turn golden brown in a few spots, 6 to 8 minutes. Push the vegetables to the outer edges of the pan and add the remaining 1 tablespoon oil. Add the cumin, sweet paprika (if using), black pepper, salt, and smoked paprika and cook, stirring occasionally, until the spices are very fragrant, 2 to 3 minutes. Add the tomato paste and cook, stirring occasionally, until caramelized to a brick red color, 4 to 5 minutes. Stir in the vinegar and scrape up the browned bits from the bottom of the pan while mixing all the ingredients together. Cook, stirring occasionally, until the vegetables are soft, about 5 minutes. Remove the skillet from the heat.

With a potato masher or large fork, mash the vegetables into a chunky sauce (some whole chunks of bell pepper will remain).

Divide the sauce between the pita rounds, spreading it over the tops. Divide the crushed walnuts between the pitas, sprinkling over the sauce. Bake for 5 minutes or until warm. Sprinkle each pita with chopped parsley and serve. Reheat any leftovers in a toaster oven.

Healthy Kitchen Hack: Tomato paste is one of our must-have pantry staples as it adds meaty, umami flavor to many soups, stews, and sauces, as we've highlighted with this recipe. If you use it often, the tubed versions are super convenient and can be stored in your refrigerator. But if you are like us and might "lose" it in the fridge, keep the canned versions on hand as they have a longer shelf life. Since you'll rarely use the entire can in one recipe, spoon the remaining paste by tablespoons into ice cube trays or onto parchment paper. Freeze and then pop the frozen dollops into a freezer-safe container for future recipes—they'll defrost quickly when mixed into whatever you're cooking!

Per Serving (2 flatbreads): Calories: 418; Total Fat: 21g; Saturated Fat: 3g; Cholesterol: 0mg; Sodium: 475mg; Total Carbohydrates: 52g; Fiber: 8g; Protein: 11g

Pear, Gorgonzola, and Roasted Kale Pita Pizzas

SERVES 4
Prep time: 10 minutes
Cook time: 20 minutes

3 ounces kale (about 3 cups), leaves and stems, sliced into ¼-inch ribbons

1 tablespoon plus 2 teaspoons extra-virgin olive oil, divided

¼ teaspoon kosher or sea salt

¼ teaspoon black pepper

1 pear

4 whole-wheat pita breads

3 ounces Gorgonzola cheese, crumbled

1 lemon

We're pretty sure you'll find yourself sneaking a few toasty, crispy shreds of kale off these pita pizzas before they get to the table—it's *that* good on its own. Kale is a great pizza topping when matched with sweet pears, tangy Gorgonzola, and tart lemon. These fall/winter "pitzas" come together quickly, and baking them in a toaster oven uses a third to half the power of a regular oven.

Preheat the toaster oven to 425°F or a regular oven to 400°F.

In a medium bowl, combine the (well-dried) kale, 2 teaspoons oil, salt, and pepper and massage, using your hands or tongs, until the kale is fully coated. Set aside for at least 5 minutes to allow the oil to soften the kale.

Cut the pear lengthwise into very thin slices. (You can remove the core or cut whole slices with the core intact—they look pretty.) Remove the stem and any seeds from the slices.

Brush the remaining 1 tablespoon oil evenly over the pita breads. Spread the pear slices over each "pitza" and top each with an even layer of sliced kale. Cook two at a time on the toaster oven tray (or all four at once on a rimmed baking sheet in a regular oven) for 10 to 12 minutes, until the kale is toasted and crispy. Remove from the oven and top with half of the cheese. Return to the oven for about 1 minute, until the cheese is melted.

Using a Microplane or citrus zester, grate the zest from the lemon over the pizzas. Cut the lemon in half and squeeze 1 tablespoon juice over the pizzas. (Save the remaining lemon juice for another use.) Serve immediately.

Healthy Kitchen Hack: To make the best kale chips, use that energy-efficient toaster oven! Preheat the toaster oven to 425°F. Line the toaster oven tray with parchment paper. Tear 1½ cups kale leaves into chip-size pieces. (Save the more tender stems to add crunch to salads or

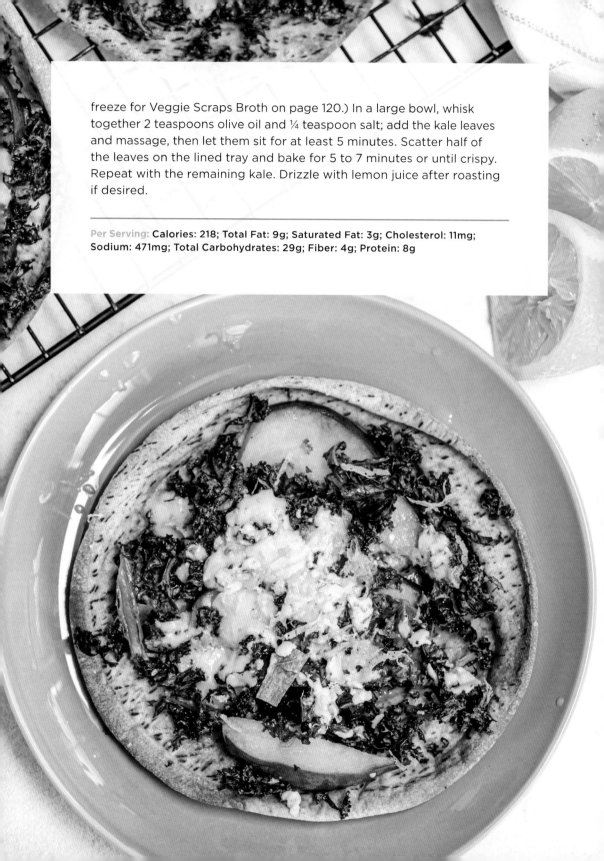

freeze for Veggie Scraps Broth on page 120.) In a large bowl, whisk together 2 teaspoons olive oil and ¼ teaspoon salt; add the kale leaves and massage, then let them sit for at least 5 minutes. Scatter half of the leaves on the lined tray and bake for 5 to 7 minutes or until crispy. Repeat with the remaining kale. Drizzle with lemon juice after roasting if desired.

Per Serving: **Calories: 218; Total Fat: 9g; Saturated Fat: 3g; Cholesterol: 11mg; Sodium: 471mg; Total Carbohydrates: 29g; Fiber: 4g; Protein: 8g**

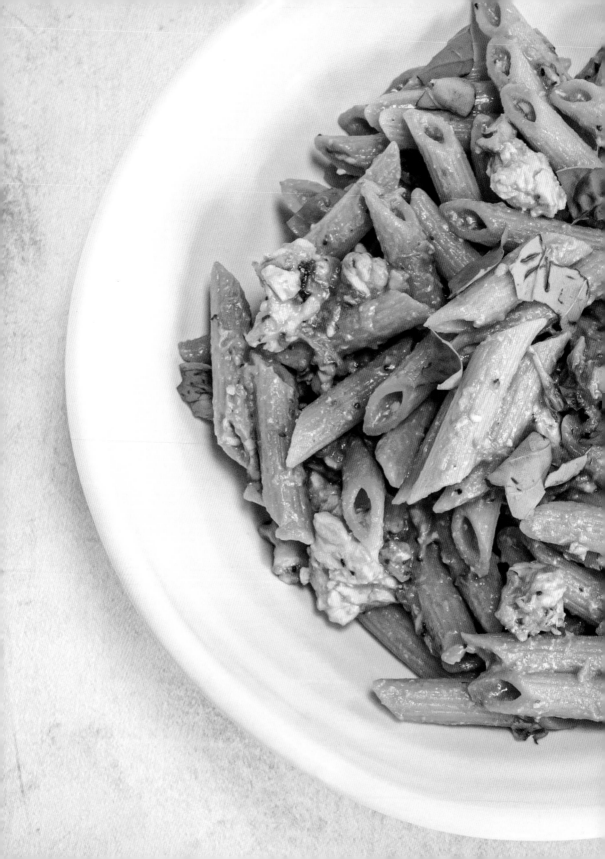

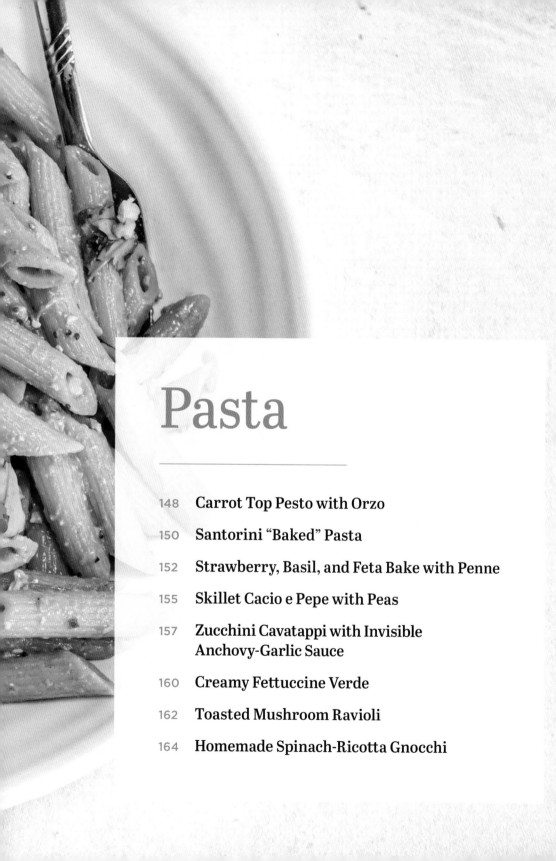

Pasta

Carrot Top Pesto with Orzo

SERVES 8
Prep time: 10 minutes
Cook time: 10 minutes

1¾ teaspoons kosher or sea salt, divided

1 (1-pound) package orzo

1 cup coarsely chopped carrot top greens, trimmed of tougher lower stems

1 cup packed spinach or fresh basil leaves and stems

¼ cup chopped peanuts

5 tablespoons grated Parmesan cheese, divided

1 garlic clove, peeled

¼ teaspoon black pepper

¼ cup extra-virgin olive oil

Home cooks often toss the leafy green stalks of root veggies like carrots, beets, and turnips (and that's assuming those cooks even brought them home, since it's common for stores to sell those vegetables without their tops). But those greens are nutritious—carrot tops have six times more vitamin C than the roots!—and they can stand in for herbs in a variety of recipes. Change your mindset and seek out vegetables with their stems still on to get the most out of the ingredients you buy. This super delish and budget-friendly pesto features carrot tops (which keep the pesto bright green!) and peanuts, a rotation crop that's an important part of sustainable farming. We like to pair this pesto with orzo, one of the quicker cooking pasta shapes.

In a large stockpot, bring 10 to 12 cups water to a boil over high heat. Add 1½ teaspoons salt and then stir in the orzo. Cook, stirring occasionally, until al dente according to the package instructions. Using a glass measuring cup, carefully scoop out about ½ cup pasta water and set it aside. Drain the orzo and transfer it to a large serving bowl. Mix in about ¼ cup pasta water, reserving the rest if needed to thin out the sauce further.

While the pasta cooks, pulse the carrot tops, spinach, peanuts, 3 tablespoons Parmesan cheese, garlic, remaining ¼ teaspoon salt, and pepper in a high-powered blender or food processor until a roughly chopped pesto forms. Scrape down the sides with a silicone scraper. With the motor running, slowly drizzle in the oil and process until smooth.

Gently stir the pesto into the serving bowl with the orzo, adding more reserved pasta water if the sauce is too thick, 1 tablespoon at a time. Sprinkle with the remaining 2 tablespoons Parmesan cheese and serve immediately.

Healthy Kitchen Hack: Make a double batch of pesto and freeze it! Spoon 1-tablespoon portions into each slot of an ice cube tray and freeze. Once frozen, transfer them to a freezer-safe container. To defrost, simply add frozen pesto cubes to hot pasta or soup and mix. To defrost as a spread, microwave in 10-second increments until thawed.

Per Serving: Calories: 313; Total Fat: 11g; Saturated Fat: 2g; Cholesterol: 2mg; Sodium: 231mg; Total Carbohydrates: 44g; Fiber: 3g; Protein: 10g

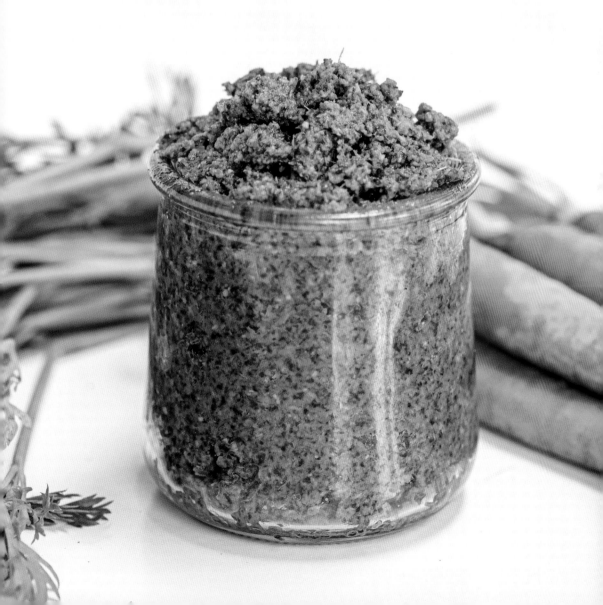

Santorini "Baked" Pasta

SERVES 8
Prep time: 20 minutes
Cook time: 15 minutes

2 teaspoons kosher or sea salt, divided

1 (1-pound) package penne

1 (14.5-ounce) can low-sodium diced tomatoes, undrained

2 cups halved cherry tomatoes, chopped tomatoes, or canned and drained diced tomatoes, divided

1 small red bell pepper, seeded and chopped

2 tablespoons capers, drained, divided

2 garlic cloves, peeled

1 tablespoon red wine vinegar

½ teaspoon crushed red pepper

¼ teaspoon black pepper

2 tablespoons extra-virgin olive oil

¾ cup shredded mozzarella or crumbled goat cheese (about 4 ounces)

Serena spent her honeymoon on the gorgeous Greek island of Santorini, which is actually a submerged volcano that's still active! The rich volcanic soils contribute to the beauty and flavor of the popular Santorini tomatoes. When you bite into one, you're hit with a rare combination of high-acid and high-sugar content that delivers a surprising tart, sweet taste. Santorini is also known for its capers, and island residents forage these plant buds and then add them, brined, to tomato salads and pasta. It's in this spirit of sustainability that we created this pasta dish with several eco-friendly cooking hacks, like a no-cook sauce (using your favorite canned tomatoes), speedier pasta boiling, and a quick oven broil (instead of baking) to make this a faster weeknight meal, all while you dream of the Greek isles.

Arrange the top oven rack about 4 inches under the broiler. Preheat the broiler to high. Coat a 2-quart broiler-safe baking dish with cooking spray.

Fill a large stockpot with 10 to 12 cups water. Cover and bring to a boil over high heat (see our quick-boil Hack following this recipe). Add 1½ teaspoons salt and then stir in the pasta. Cook, stirring occasionally, for 1 to 2 minutes short of al dente according to the package instructions. Drain the pasta and transfer to the prepared baking dish.

While the pasta cooks, in a food processor or blender, puree the canned tomatoes with their juices, 1 cup cherry tomatoes, bell pepper, 1 tablespoon capers, garlic, vinegar, remaining ½ teaspoon salt, crushed red pepper, and black pepper. With the motor running, pour in the olive oil and process until smooth.

Pour the tomato mixture over the pasta in the baking dish and add the remaining 1 cup cherry tomatoes and remaining 1 tablespoon capers; stir well. Sprinkle the cheese over the top. Broil for about 3 minutes or until the mozzarella cheese just starts to turn golden brown or the goat cheese softens.

Healthy Kitchen Hack: We tend to be minimalists in the kitchen, using fewer gadgets and utensils. But if you want to lower your electricity use when it comes to boiling water, consider purchasing an electric water kettle (look for used options at online resale groups). Serena uses hers daily for boiling water for oatmeal, instant coffee, and tea, for quickly thawing frozen vegetables and berries, and for pasta water. Boiling a big pot of water to cook pasta (4 to 6 quarts is typically recommended on the package) can take up to 15 minutes. But to minimize energy and water use, use only 3 quarts (12 cups) water and boil some of it in the quicker-heating electric kettle. Boil 2 quarts (8 cups) water in the electric kettle while also boiling 1 quart (4 cups) in your pot on the stove, then dump the boiling kettle water into the pot. This whole process takes only 6 minutes. (Yes, Serena timed it!)

Per Serving: Calories: 304; Total Fat: 6g; Saturated Fat: 1.6g; Cholesterol: 5mg; Sodium: 377mg; Total Carbohydrates: 50g; Fiber: 4g; Protein: 12g

Strawberry, Basil, and Feta Bake with Penne

SERVES 8
Prep time: 10 minutes
Cook time: 35 minutes

2 pounds fresh strawberries (about 35), hulled and quartered (see Hack)

3 tablespoons extra-virgin olive oil, divided

1 (8-ounce) block feta cheese, removed from brine

½ teaspoon black pepper, divided

1½ teaspoons kosher or sea salt

1 (1-pound) package penne

1 cup fresh basil leaves, gently torn

4 teaspoons balsamic vinegar (optional)

Before you pause at the thought of baked strawberries paired with tangy cheese, remember that tomatoes (a classic pasta and cheese pairing) are actually a fruit, too! In fact, full credit for this fabulous dish goes to our dietetic student intern, Kennedy, who took the TikTok-famed Baked Feta Pasta recipe and gave it this unique and delectable twist—perfect for strawberry season! You can even skip the penne altogether, serving the warm feta straight out of the oven as a fun appetizer with pita wedges for dipping.

Preheat the oven to 425°F.

In a 9 × 13-inch baking dish, toss together the strawberries and 2 tablespoons oil using your hands or a spoon. Place the block of feta in the center of the dish, making sure there are no strawberries under the feta, only surrounding it. Drizzle the remaining 1 tablespoon oil over the feta and sprinkle with ¼ teaspoon pepper. Bake for 30 to 35 minutes or until the feta turns light brown and the strawberries are soft and bubbling in their juices.

Meanwhile, fill a large stockpot with 10 to 12 cups water. Cover and bring to a boil over high heat. Add the salt and then stir in the penne. Cook, stirring occasionally, until al dente according to the package instructions. Using a glass measuring cup, carefully scoop out about ½ cup pasta water, then set aside. Drain the pasta and return it to the warm pot.

When ready to serve, break up the feta with a wooden spoon and mix gently with the cooked strawberries. Add the pasta and stir all the ingredients together (see how the served version looks on page 146). To make a slightly thick sauce, stir in the reserved pasta water, 1 tablespoon at a time, if needed. Sprinkle with the basil and remaining ¼ teaspoon pepper, and drizzle with balsamic vinegar if desired.

Healthy Kitchen Hack: Instead of slicing off the tops of your strawberries to remove the green hulls (along with part of the edible flesh, too), use a reusable metal or bamboo straw. Gently insert the straw through the bottom middle of the strawberry and guide it to come out the top end, popping off the green leaves of the hull. You can even add the hulls to a pitcher of water (for up to 2 days in the fridge) to give your drink a lovely essence of strawberry!

Per Serving: Calories: 371; Total Fat: 13g; Saturated Fat: 5g; Cholesterol: 25mg; Sodium: 296mg; Total Carbohydrates: 53g; Fiber: 4g; Protein: 12g

"This is such a unique yet easy dish to make. The strawberries make it so pretty, it would be lovely as a dip or even a meal for Valentine's Day or a baby or bridal shower."

—Jamie from San Jose, CA

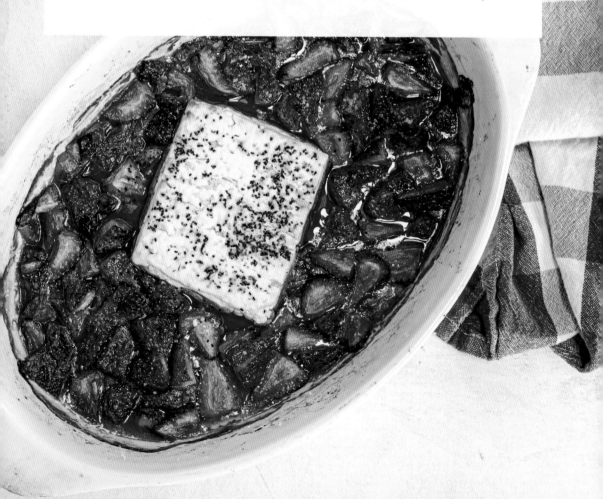

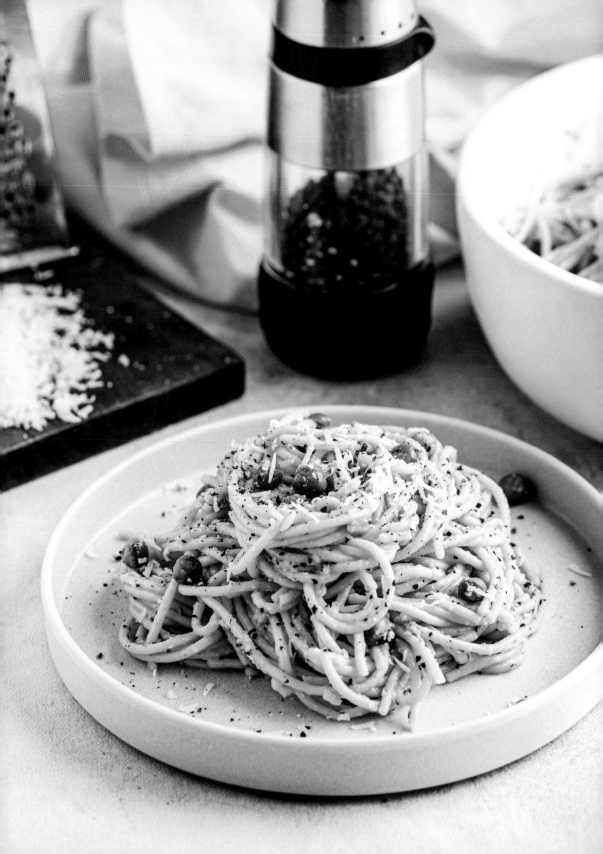

Skillet Cacio e Pepe with Peas

SERVES 4
Prep time: 15 minutes
Cook time: 20 minutes

1 cup frozen peas

1½ teaspoons kosher or sea salt

½ (1-pound) package spaghetti or linguine

4 teaspoons extra-virgin olive oil

2 teaspoons freshly ground black pepper, plus more for serving if desired

¾ cup freshly grated Parmesan cheese (about 2 ounces)

In Italian, *cacio e pepe* simply means cheese and pepper. But don't mistake simple for boring—this black pepper–infused pasta is anything but! Besides the intense flavor, we also like that the starchy, salty pasta water becomes part of the recipe, so a smaller amount of water is needed to initially cook the pasta. Also, some of the cooking occurs off the stove, using the warm pasta water to thaw the peas and melt the cheese, which means less energy is used compared to other classic pasta recipes. For the most satisfying results, take the extra few minutes to freshly grind the black pepper and grate the cheese.

Put the frozen peas in a large serving bowl so they can start to thaw as you make the pasta.

Fill a large stockpot with 8 cups water. Cover and bring to a boil over high heat. Add the salt and then stir in the pasta. Cook, stirring occasionally, for 1 to 2 minutes short of al dente according to the package instructions. Using tongs, transfer the pasta to the serving bowl with the peas; reserve the pasta cooking water in the pot.

While the pasta cooks, heat the oil in a small skillet over medium heat. Add the pepper and cook, stirring once, until very fragrant and just starting to sizzle, 2 to 3 minutes. (Be careful not to burn the pepper.) Remove from the heat and let the skillet cool for 5 minutes to prevent the oil from splattering in the next step.

Return the skillet to the stove, turn the heat up to medium-high, and add 1 cup reserved pasta water. Cook until about ¾ cup water remains (eyeball it in the pan), about 5 minutes. Pour this pepper mixture over the pasta and peas in the serving bowl. Using two forks or tongs, toss the pasta to coat it well until almost all the liquid is absorbed (except about ¼ cup—again, eyeball it), at least 3 minutes. (This is a key step to coat the pasta.) Add ¼ cup cheese and 2 more tablespoons reserved pasta water and toss well for at least another minute. Repeat this step with an additional ¼ cup cheese; toss well until the pasta is coated and almost all the liquid is absorbed.

continued

Skillet Cacio e Pepe with Peas *(continued)*

Top the pasta with the remaining ¼ cup cheese and additional freshly ground black pepper if desired. Serve immediately.

Healthy Kitchen Hack: We "heart" freshly ground black pepper and encourage you to purchase a pepper mill and then fill it with peppercorns. While this can make measuring seem challenging, here's what we do: grind 15 turns of a pepper mill onto parchment paper, then form the paper into a funnel and pour the pepper into a measuring spoon (it will probably be around ¼ teaspoon). Make note if your mill makes a similar amount (or adjust by more or fewer grinds to get close to ¼ teaspoon), then each time you need ¼ teaspoon of pepper, simply grind that many times, or multiply the number of pepper grinds for a larger measurement.

Per Serving: Calories: 338; Total Fat: 10g; Saturated Fat: 3g; Cholesterol: 10mg; Sodium: 473mg; Total Carbohydrates: 48g; Fiber: 4g; Protein: 15g

Zucchini Cavatappi with Invisible Anchovy-Garlic Sauce

SERVES 4
Prep time: 15 minutes
Cook time: 20 minutes

1½ teaspoons kosher or sea salt

½ (1-pound) package cavatappi or other medium-size pasta, like penne, fusilli, or orecchiette

1 (2-ounce) tin anchovies in olive oil, undrained

2 tablespoons extra-virgin olive oil

4 garlic cloves, minced

¼ teaspoon crushed red pepper, plus more for serving if desired

4 large, 5 medium, or 6 small zucchini, finely chopped (about 6 cups)

1 batch Made-in-Minutes Homemade Ricotta Cheese (page 48) plus 1 tablespoon of the whey *or* ¾ cup store-bought whole-milk ricotta cheese, plus more for serving if desired

¼ teaspoon black pepper

½ cup shaved Parmesan or Pecorino Romano cheese (about 2 ounces)

Anchovies often get a bad rap with that "right-in-your-face" aroma. But they are truly the ultimate savory flavor enhancer (check out Deanna's Zesty Garlic Sauce on page 100 if you haven't already!). And when cooked correctly, they can deliver incredible, non-fishy umami, as in this easy pot of pasta. The anchovies will break apart and seem to "melt" into a garlicky, peppery sauce that pairs well with mild zucchini—we doubt anyone will detect any fish in this dish! Be sure to make it during summer squash season; you'll use up several zucchini here.

Fill a large stockpot with 10 to 12 cups water. Cover and bring to a boil over high heat. Add the salt and then stir in the cavatappi. Cook, stirring occasionally, until al dente according to the package instructions. Using a glass measuring cup, carefully scoop out about ½ cup pasta water, then set aside. Drain the pasta and transfer it to a large serving bowl.

While the pasta cooks, using a fork, remove the anchovies from the tin and set aside. Heat the oil from the anchovy tin and the olive oil in a large saucepan or Dutch oven over medium heat. Add the anchovies, garlic, and crushed red pepper and cook for 2 minutes, stirring frequently and mashing up the anchovies with the back of your spoon or spatula, until well mixed. Add the zucchini and stir until all the pieces are coated in the seasoned oil. Cover and cook, lifting the lid and stirring every few minutes, until the zucchini pieces cook down into the sauce, at least 15 minutes. (Note: the zucchini will release a lot of liquid, so stirring occasionally will help create a more cohesive sauce.)

Once the pasta is done, remove the zucchini from the heat and gently mix in the ricotta and black pepper. Depending on your sauce preference (thicker or thinner), mix in 1 to 3 tablespoons reserved pasta water. Pour the skillet sauce over the hot pasta. Add the shaved cheese

continued

and gently mix until well incorporated. Serve immediately, with extra ricotta and/or crushed red pepper for topping if desired.

Healthy Kitchen Hack: Made a recipe that calls for only a few anchovy fillets? Don't let the leftovers be forgotten in your fridge! Here are some other yummy ideas for what to do with anchovies: whisk into a dressing for our Roasted Cabbage Wedge Caesar Salad (page 78); chop and mix into chili, stews, or tomato-based soups; or smash and cook into a tomato sauce. Or use them in our Lemon Charred Asparagus (page 100) or Creamy Chicken Skillet Supper with Greens (page 251).

Per Serving: Calories: 446; Total Fat: 19g; Saturated Fat: 7g; Cholesterol: 46mg; Sodium: 740mg; Total Carbohydrates: 48g; Fiber: 2g; Protein: 21g

"This is such a great way to use up zucchini and to incorporate more veggies! I never thought to use zucchini in a pasta sauce. And I would have never known there were anchovies in the sauce."

—Rachel from Saint Paul, MN

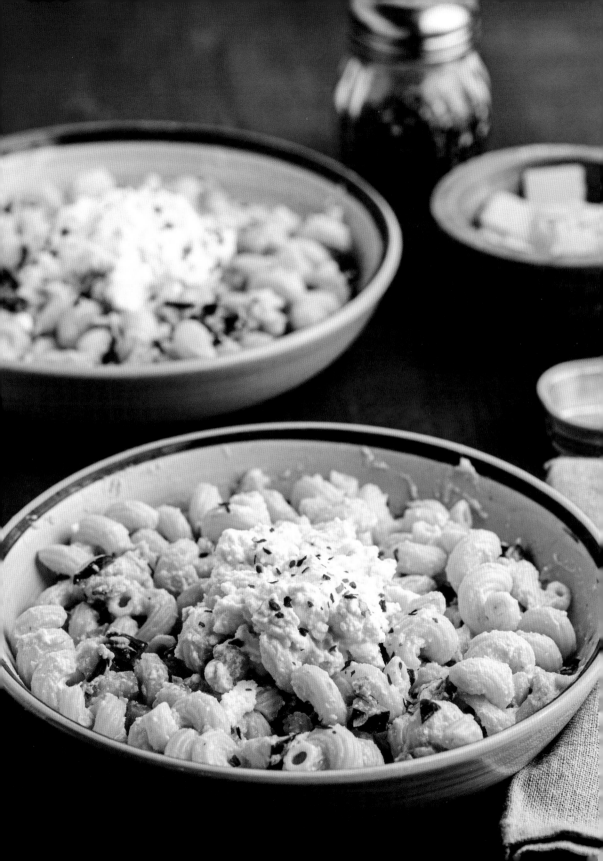

Creamy Fettuccine Verde

SERVES 6
Prep time: 5 minutes
Cook time: 15 minutes

2 teaspoons kosher or sea salt, divided

1 (1-pound) package fettuccine

1 lemon

2 cups chopped fresh cilantro or parsley, leaves and stems, divided

1½ cups plain 2% Greek yogurt

3 large egg yolks
Save the whites to make scrambled eggs or an omelet

1 garlic clove, peeled

½ cup grated Parmesan cheese

½ teaspoon black pepper

Birthdays at the Ball household are highly anticipated for their gift surprises, but the celebratory meal itself is never a surprise. Year after year, it's always a big pot of fettuccine carbonara, the classic Italian pasta dish in a sauce of egg yolks, cheese, cured meat, and lots of black pepper. Serena took her family's favorite and made it "green"—both in color and by implementing several of our sustainability strategies, such as boiling the fettuccine in less water, incorporating some of the pasta water into the sauce, and using the cilantro leaves *and* stems. Her surprise twist is blending in plain Greek yogurt, which effortlessly pulls the entire recipe together. Make this meal your own by adding favorite pantry staples like canned chickpeas or roasted red peppers or by using up leftovers in the fridge such as cooked sausage or chicken. Or, just enjoy a big satisfying bowl of noodles any weeknight, even if there's no birthday to celebrate.

Fill a large stockpot with 10 to 12 cups water. Cover and bring to a boil over high heat. Add 1½ teaspoons salt and then stir in the fettuccine. Cook, stirring occasionally, until al dente according to the package instructions. Using a glass measuring cup, carefully scoop out about ½ cup pasta water and set it aside. Drain the pasta and return it to the warm pot.

While the pasta cooks, using a Microplane or citrus zester, grate the zest from the lemon over a blender; set the lemon aside. To the blender, add the cilantro, yogurt, egg yolks, garlic, and the remaining ½ teaspoon salt; puree until smooth.

Pour the blender mixture over the pasta and cook over medium heat, stirring constantly, until the sauce thickens and coats the pasta, about 3 minutes. (You may not need the reserved pasta cooking water, but if you want your sauce more liquidy or if your pasta has cooled, mix in a couple tablespoons to help the sauce coat the noodles.) Remove the pot from the heat. Cut the lemon in half and squeeze in the juice from one half. Add the cheese and pepper and stir to combine. Cut the other lemon half into wedges and serve with the warm pasta.

Healthy Kitchen Hack: Don't dump that reserved "liquid gold" pasta cooking water! Store it in a jar in the fridge. It works wonders when heating up pasta leftovers, whether they are plain noodles or a baked pasta dish. Use the classic restaurant kitchen trick of adding a few tablespoons of the pasta water if warming noodles on the stove or in the microwave. The starchy water will help restore it to a closer resemblance of freshly cooked pasta while ensuring the sauce will stick.

Per Serving: Calories: 375; Total Fat: 6g; Saturated Fat: 2g; Cholesterol: 100mg; Sodium: 286mg; Total Carbohydrates: 62g; Fiber: 3g; Protein: 19g

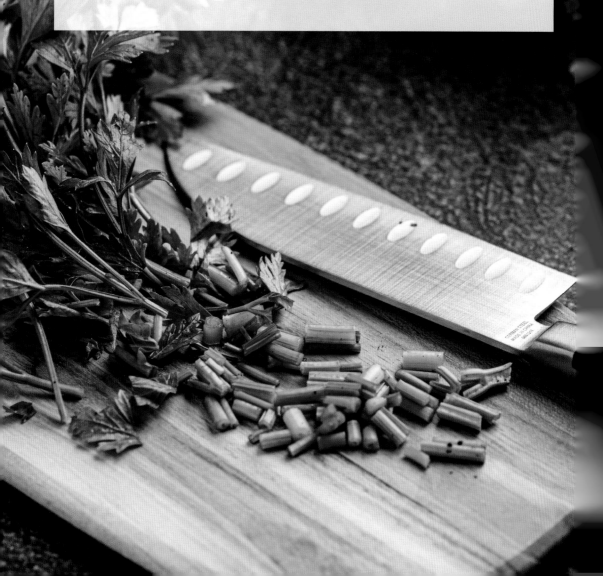

Toasted Mushroom Ravioli

SERVES 6
Prep time: 20 minutes
Cook time: 25 minutes

1 tablespoon extra-virgin olive oil

1 pound mushrooms (any type), finely chopped

3 garlic cloves, minced

1 tablespoon dried oregano

¼ teaspoon kosher or sea salt

¼ teaspoon black pepper

1 tablespoon balsamic vinegar

1 batch Made-in-Minutes Homemade Ricotta Cheese (page 48) *or* ¾ cup store-bought whole-milk ricotta cheese

1 (12-ounce) package wonton wrappers

½ (24-ounce) jar low-sodium tomato pasta sauce

Near where Serena lives in Saint Louis, the specialty appetizer at many Italian American restaurants is toasted ravioli: crispy, deep-fried, meat-filled ravioli with a side of marinara sauce for dipping. But they aren't exactly authentic Mediterranean diet food. So, we baked and "veggie-fied" them by stuffing with hearty mushrooms, a staple ingredient from everywhere in the "boot" of Italy from the heel to the toe! Of course, mushrooms are grown in the US, too, and they are one of the most sustainable vegetables as well as being super rich in nutrients. And even mushroom detractors (like Serena's kids) will likely devour this vegetarian version of "t-ravs." Round out the meal by serving a salad (topped with oven-crisped leftover wonton wrapper croutons) and crusty whole-grain bread.

Arrange the oven racks to the upper-middle and lower-middle positions. Preheat the oven to 375°F. Coat two large rimmed baking sheets with cooking spray.

Heat the oil in a large skillet over medium heat. Add the mushrooms, garlic, oregano, salt, and pepper. Turn the heat up to medium-high and cook, stirring frequently, until the mushrooms are slightly wilted, about 5 minutes. Add the vinegar and cook, stirring frequently, until the liquid has evaporated, 3 to 5 minutes. Transfer the mushroom mixture to a medium bowl, add the ricotta cheese, and mix well.

Fill a small bowl with water and put it near your work surface. Place one wonton wrapper on a dry surface. (Keep the remaining wonton wrappers in the package while you work so they don't dry out.) Add 1½ teaspoons mushroom filling to the center of the wonton. Dip your finger in the water and run it along two sides of the wonton wrapper (to make the wrapper sticky). Fold the wonton wrapper over, matching two corners to make a triangle, then press the sides together to seal. Place the sealed ravioli on the prepared baking sheets. Repeat with the remaining wonton wrappers and filling, placing no more than 18 ravioli on each baking sheet. (If the ravioli are crowded, they won't crisp.) Coat the tops of the ravioli with cooking spray. Bake for 6 minutes, then turn over each ravioli and swap the positions of the baking sheets on the oven racks. Bake for an additional 5 to 7 minutes, until the edges are deep golden. Transfer the ravioli to a serving platter.

Serve with tomato sauce.

Healthy Kitchen Hack: Got mushrooms? If you don't have fresh white, cremini, wild, or foraged mushrooms, take advantage of another one of our favorite pantry staples: canned mushrooms! Drain (reserving the liquid) and rinse. Replace the small bowl of water you use to seal the wontons with some of the mushroom liquid. Or if you have leftover Roasted Thyme Mushrooms from our recipe on page 193, they'd work well here, too.

Per Serving: Calories: 220; Total Fat: 7g; Saturated Fat: 3g; Cholesterol: 16mg; Sodium: 431mg; Total Carbohydrates: 31g; Fiber: 2g; Protein: 11g

Homemade Spinach-Ricotta Gnocchi

SERVES 4
Prep time: 15 minutes
Cook time: 15 minutes

1 (1-pound) bag frozen chopped spinach

2 batches Made-in-Minutes Ricotta Cheese (page 48) *or* 1½ cups store-bought part-skim ricotta cheese

¾ cup all-purpose flour

8 tablespoons grated Parmesan cheese, divided

2 large egg yolks

½ teaspoon ground nutmeg

½ teaspoon kosher or sea salt

1 cup your favorite canned or jarred low-sodium tomato sauce

"I couldn't believe how light and fluffy these were— so much better than the dense version you can buy at the store."

—Flavio from
Silver Spring, MD

If you've never made homemade pasta before, this recipe for pillowy ricotta-based gnocchi will change all that. Unlike potato gnocchi (which Deanna's Italian American Pop-Pop used to call "sinkers" because of their density), these light-as-air gnocchi feature convenient frozen spinach and just enough flour to hold their easy-to-make, larger meatball shape together while cooking. Fresh pasta cooks up in less than half the time of its dried counterpart, which means less energy to heat the water and no packaging waste. Speaking of no waste—don't toss those egg whites! While this recipe calls for just yolks, save the whites to add to scrambled eggs or an omelet, or for your next batch of cookies. If you don't need to keep this dish vegetarian, serve with our Savory Sardine Tomato Sauce (page 210).

Empty the frozen spinach into a large microwave-safe bowl. Microwave on high for 3 minutes, then stir and microwave for an additional 1 to 1½ minutes or until thawed. Transfer the spinach to a clean tea towel and wring out as much liquid as possible over the sink. Pat the spinach dry with another towel.

Wipe out the bowl and return the spinach to it. Add the ricotta, flour, 3 tablespoons Parmesan cheese, egg yolks, nutmeg, and salt. Using a wooden spoon or your hands, mix together well until a soft, sticky dough forms. Using a measuring spoon, scoop 1 tablespoon dough and form a ball. Transfer to a baking sheet and repeat the process to make about 32 gnocchi.

Fill a large stockpot with 8 cups water and bring to a gentle boil. Carefully drop half of the gnocchi into the water and cook until they rise to the top, about 4 minutes. Using a slotted spoon, skimmer, or kitchen spider, gently remove the gnocchi and transfer to a serving bowl. Repeat with the remaining gnocchi. Top with the tomato sauce and remaining Parmesan cheese and serve.

Healthy Kitchen Hack: The key to making these light gnocchi stay together and not fall apart when cooking is to remove as much moisture as possible from the dough ingredients. Cooked spinach retains *a lot* of liquid, so give that tea towel a few more squeezes even after you think you've gotten rid of every drop. And if you have time, drain store-bought ricotta through a fine-mesh strainer for 15 minutes to remove even more liquid (save it to mix into oatmeal, pancake batter, or smoothies). If you use our Made-in-Minutes Homemade Ricotta, draining is unnecessary because it is lower in moisture than store-bought.

Per Serving (8 gnocchi): Calories: 288; Total Fat: 12g; Saturated Fat: 6g; Cholesterol: 125mg; Sodium: 391mg; Total Carbohydrates: 28g; Fiber: 3g; Protein: 19g

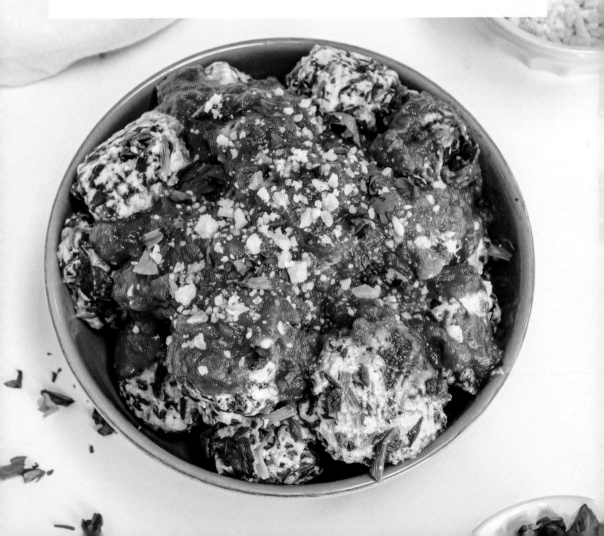

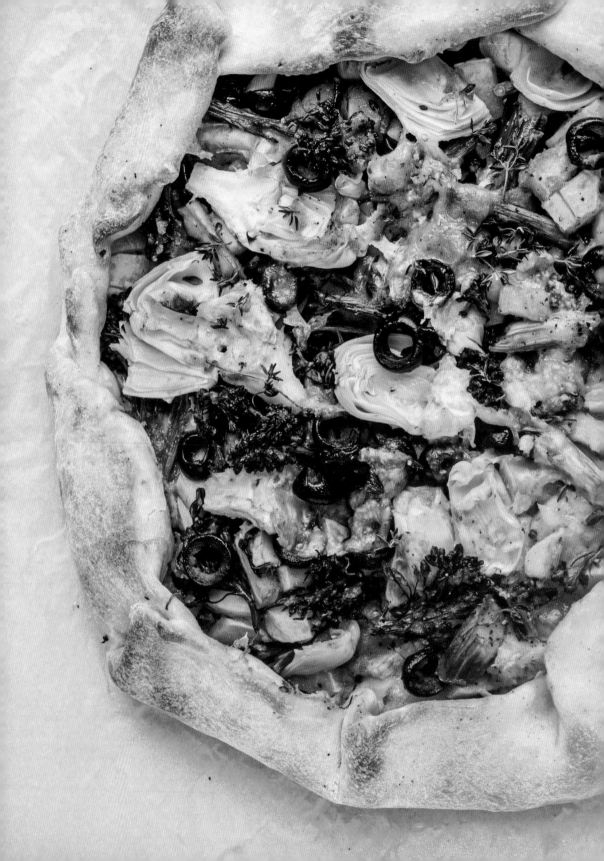

Vegetarian Main Dishes

Slow Cooker Red Pepper and Eggplant Parmesan

SERVES 6

Prep time: 15 minutes
Cook time: 8 hours

2 large eggs

¼ cup 2% milk

1 cup panko or regular bread crumbs

⅓ cup grated Parmesan or Pecorino Romano cheese (about 1½ ounces), divided

¼ teaspoon black pepper

1 (1-pound) globe eggplant, stemmed and cut into ½-inch rounds

1 (28-ounce) can or jar low-sodium marinara or tomato sauce

3 red bell peppers, seeded and cut into 2-inch strips

2 cups shredded mozzarella cheese (about 8 ounces)

¼ cup fresh basil leaves (8 to 10 leaves), torn

We're always up for the challenge of converting eggplant dislikers into eggplant embracers (Serena, at one time, was in the former camp). And we get it—when eggplant isn't cooked correctly, it can be rubbery and tasteless. But with this version of the classic Italian dish, your slow cooker becomes eggplant's best friend, resulting in a silky-smooth, cheesy, melt-in-your-mouth meal. Make this during the summer when peppers and eggplant are abundant at local markets (or perhaps even from your own garden!), and use that energy-saving slow cooker to avoid heating up the kitchen with a hot oven.

In a large, shallow bowl, whisk together the eggs and milk. In another large shallow bowl, mix together the panko, ¼ cup Parmesan cheese, and black pepper. Dip each eggplant slice into the egg mixture, coating both sides, and then into the panko-cheese coating, again coating both sides. Place the breaded slices on a plate.

Pour a thin layer of marinara sauce into a 6-quart slow cooker. To start the layering process, lay one-third of the eggplant slices over the sauce, slightly overlapping each slice. Layer in one-third of the pepper slices. Cover with one-third of the remaining sauce. Sprinkle ⅔ cup mozzarella cheese over the top. Repeat the layering process two more times.

Cover and cook on high for 4 hours or on low for 8 hours, until the sauce is bubbly and the peppers are completely soft. When serving, sprinkle each portion with the remaining Parmesan cheese and torn basil.

Healthy Kitchen Hack: Though it's not a Mediterranean staple ingredient, we prefer using panko (and whole-wheat panko when we can find it) for recipes that call for bread crumbs. This Japanese style of bread crumbs are dried as flakes instead of crumbs, which results in a crispier and lighter texture when coating and cooking foods, using less oil. That said, in this recipe, using panko doesn't matter as much because the eggplant is baked slowly instead of being sautéed or fried, so use whatever you have on hand. For a gluten-free option, try stone-ground cornmeal for coating instead.

Per Serving: Calories: 333; Total Fat: 13g; Saturated Fat: 6g; Cholesterol: 93mg; Sodium: 524mg; Total Carbohydrates: 36g; Fiber: 8g; Protein: 20g

"I really liked this version of eggplant parm. My husband even enjoyed it—and he rarely eats eggplant!"

—Suzanne from Litchfield, IL

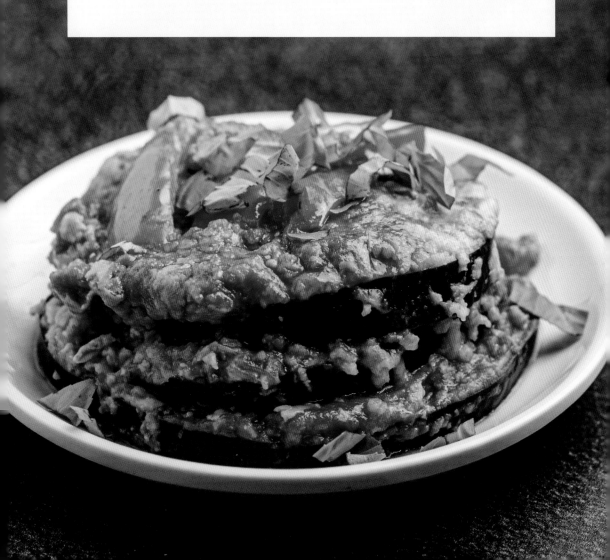

Everyday Pot of Lentils

SERVES 8
Prep time: 10 minutes
Cook time: 15 minutes

- 2 tablespoons extra-virgin olive oil
- 1 medium onion (any type), chopped
- 2 garlic cloves, minced
- 2 tablespoons tomato paste
- 2 cups dried brown lentils
- 2 thyme sprigs
- ½ teaspoon kosher or sea salt
- ¼ cup chopped fresh parsley, leaves and stems
- 1 tablespoon red wine vinegar
- ¼ teaspoon black pepper

We've heard it from more than one of our Facebook Live viewers and several friends: "I don't like beans, but I'll eat lentils." So, here's our staple recipe for lentils that's so easy you could make it every day—and so tasty that you'll want to. Lentils are foundational to the health benefits of the Mediterranean lifestyle, and they're also one of the key reasons that the diet is so sustainable. Most common (and our go-to) are brown lentils, which have an outer seed coat, so they stay somewhat firm during cooking, making them perfect for salads, side dishes, and stews. Serve this perfect pot of lentils as a side dish, mixed into a bowl of whole grains like bulgur or farro, as individual bowls with a fried egg on top, or pureed into soup.

Heat the oil in a large saucepan or Dutch oven over medium heat. Add the onion, garlic, and tomato paste and cook, stirring occasionally, for 5 minutes, until fragrant. Add the lentils, thyme, salt, and 4½ cups water and bring to a boil over high heat. Reduce the heat to medium-low and simmer for about 30 minutes or until the lentils are tender but not mushy; they should still have a bit of a bite. Remove the thyme sprigs. Stir in the parsley, vinegar, and pepper.

Flavor Options

Give your lentils passports of flavor around the Mediterranean with these combinations:

North African: With the thyme, add 2 teaspoons ground cumin and 1 teaspoon ground coriander (or dried oregano). Stir in cilantro instead of parsley. Serve with cooked couscous.

Turkish: With the thyme, add 1 teaspoon smoked paprika and ½ teaspoon ground cinnamon. Stir in cilantro instead of parsley. Serve with cooked bulgur.

Greek: With the thyme, add 1 tablespoon dried oregano. Stir in dill instead of parsley. Serve with pita bread.

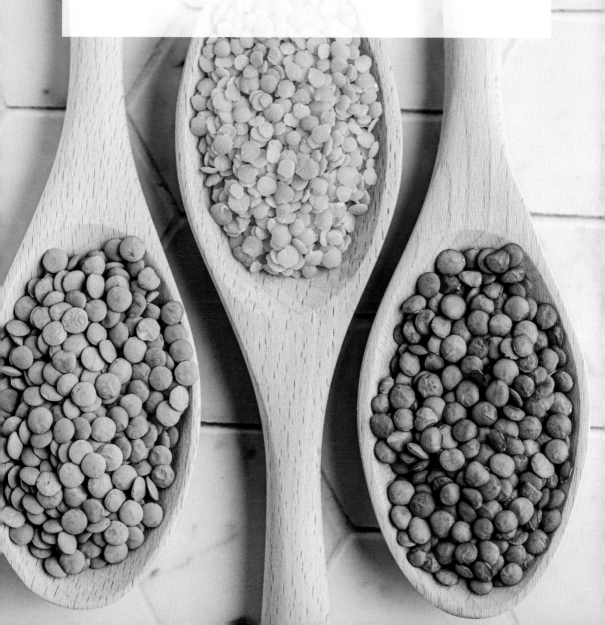

Healthy Kitchen Hack: Here's a lentil cooking formula that you can adjust: 1 cup dried rinsed lentils + 2 to 3 cups water = 2½ cups cooked lentils. If you plan to watch the lentils closely, use 2 cups water. If you don't, use 3 cups; you can always drain liquid after cooking, which is better than a dry, scorched pot that wasn't watched.

Per Serving: Calories: 212; Total Fat: 4g; Saturated Fat: 0g; Cholesterol: 0mg; Sodium: 152mg; Total Carbohydrates: 34g; Fiber: 6g; Protein: 12g

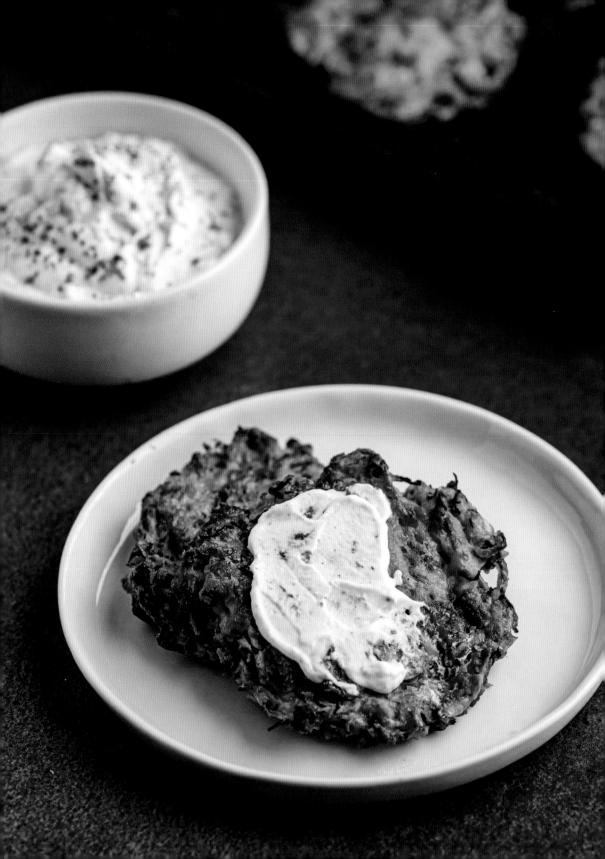

Zucchini, Carrot, and Gorgonzola Patties

SERVES 4
Prep time: 15 minutes
Cook time: 25 minutes

1 large or 2 small zucchini

1 large or 2 small carrots

4 ounces Gorgonzola or blue cheese, crumbled

½ cup chickpea flour

½ cup chopped fresh cilantro and/or parsley, leaves and stems

1 large egg

¼ teaspoon kosher or sea salt

¼ teaspoon black pepper

3 tablespoons extra-virgin olive oil, divided

1 lemon

½ cup plain 2% Greek yogurt

1 teaspoon za'atar

A riff on zucchini pancakes and potato latkes, these colorful veggie cakes are loaded with some of our favorite Mediterranean flavor bombs. Baked for a hands-off, no-splattering-oil approach, they are easy to adapt to include ingredients you need to use up, especially if you have any extra shreds from making our Tahini Use-Up-Those-Veggies Slaw (page 75). In colder months, pair these patties with one of our soups, like Vegetarian French Onion and Barley Soup (page 112); when hotter temperatures prevail, serve them over or next to a bed of leafy greens, like our Honey, Orange, and Scallion Vinaigrette over Romaine (page 70). And see this recipe's Healthy Kitchen Hack for several different variations to this satisfying plant-forward meal.

Preheat the oven to 425°F. Coat a large rimmed baking sheet with cooking spray.

Trim the ends of the zucchini (save them in your Veggie Scraps Broth freezer bag—see page 120—or compost them). Using a box grater, shred the zucchini (you should have about 1½ cups). Transfer to a clean tea towel and squeeze tightly over the sink to extract as much moisture as possible. Squeeze at least two more times (zucchini holds *a lot* of liquid). Repeat the same trim, shred, and squeeze process with the carrot (you should have about 1½ cups); since carrots have less moisture, one firm squeeze will be fine. (Note: Squeezing out excess moisture is essential to allow the fritters to crisp up in the oven.)

Dump the shredded veggies into a large bowl. Add the Gorgonzola, chickpea flour, herbs, egg, salt, and pepper. Using your hands, mix all the ingredients until everything sticks together. Using a ¼-cup scoop, shape into 12 patties. Transfer them to the prepared baking sheet and flatten with your hand to approximately ½-inch thickness. Brush the tops with 1½ tablespoons oil. Bake for 15 minutes.

continued

Remove the sheet from the oven. Flip each fritter and brush with the remaining 1½ tablespoons oil. Return the sheet to the oven and bake until the fritters are crisp and cooked through, an additional 8 to 10 minutes.

While the fritters bake, using a Microplane or citrus zester, grate the zest from the lemon over a small bowl. Cut the lemon in half and squeeze in 1 to 2 teaspoons juice (depending on how thick or thin you want the yogurt topping). Whisk in the yogurt and za'atar. Serve the yogurt topping with the warm fritters.

Healthy Kitchen Hack: Besides switching up the shredded veggies (think broccoli stems, beets, cabbage, and/or potatoes), you can swap out the green herbs for these spice combos depending on your mood and, of course, what you have on hand (that's the sustainable way!). For a sweeter version, mix in 1 teaspoon ground cinnamon and ½ teaspoon ground nutmeg, and mix 2 teaspoons honey into the yogurt topping instead of the za'atar. Or go Greek and use chopped fresh dill and/or mint and add crumbled feta instead of the Gorgonzola; then swap dried oregano for the za'atar in the yogurt and add ¼ cup diced cucumber. Or if you want to bring on the heat, stir in Serena's harissa spice blend featured on page 249 (paprika through garlic powder), then add a few pinches of crushed red pepper to the yogurt topping.

Per Serving (3 fritters): **Calories: 279; Total Fat: 21g; Saturated Fat: 8g; Cholesterol: 72mg; Sodium: 510mg; Total Carbohydrates: 13g; Fiber: 3g; Protein: 12g**

Cauliflower Steaks with Sun-Dried Tomato and Basil Pesto

SERVES 4
Prep time: 20 minutes
Cook time: 30 minutes

1 large or 2 medium heads cauliflower (see Note)

2 tablespoons extra-virgin olive oil, divided

¼ teaspoon kosher or sea salt, divided

¼ teaspoon black pepper, divided

1 lemon

1 cup chopped fresh parsley, leaves and stems

½ cup chopped fresh basil, leaves and stems

½ cup chopped walnuts or other nuts

1 garlic clove, peeled

8 sun-dried tomatoes in oil, drained and oil reserved, coarsely chopped

¼ cup shaved Parmesan cheese

While the red, white, and green color palette of this dish makes a gorgeous plate, the whole dish is very "green" as you'll employ several of our sustainability guidelines to make it. You'll use up the *whole* cauliflower, including the extra florets and crumbles from cutting and those sweeter, tender, light green leaves on the stalk. Rather than tossing the sun-dried tomato liquid down the drain, you'll whisk it into the irresistible pesto sauce. And you'll save some cooking time and energy by placing the baking sheet in the cold oven and then preheating it, which gives the cauliflower a head start in roasting when it hits the oven.

Arrange both oven racks in the top half of the oven and place two large rimmed baking sheets on them. Preheat the oven to 425°F (with the sheets inside).

With the cauliflower stem-end down, trim away all the light green leaves around the base, coarsely chop, and set aside. With a chef's knife, slice down through the center of the head, including the stem. Out of each half-head, make two ¾-inch "steaks," for a total of four steaks (see Note). Put the remaining florets and stem bits in a medium bowl. Scrape the cauliflower "crumbles" off the cutting board and add to the pile of light green leaves that have been set aside.

Pat the cauliflower steaks dry with a towel (carefully so the steaks do not fall apart), then brush 1 tablespoon oil generously over the steaks and sprinkle them with ⅛ teaspoon each salt and pepper. Pour the remaining 1 tablespoon oil over the florets and stems and toss to coat. Sprinkle with the remaining ⅛ teaspoon each salt and pepper, then toss.

Carefully remove the preheated baking sheets from the oven and coat with cooking spray. Immediately arrange the cauliflower steaks and florets on the pans so they have room for air to circulate around them.

continued

Return the sheets to the top half of the oven and roast for about 30 minutes, until the bottoms of the cauliflower steaks turn dark golden, switching the sheets' position halfway through. (Do not flip the steaks during roasting.)

While the cauliflower roasts, make the pesto. Using a Microplane or citrus zester, grate the zest from the lemon into a blender or food processor, then cut the lemon in half and squeeze in the juice. Add the reserved cauliflower green leaves and crumbles, parsley, basil, walnuts, and garlic and pulse until combined. With the blender running, pour in 3 tablespoons oil from the sun-dried tomatoes jar (save the sun-dried tomatoes for serving) and about 2 tablespoons water until the pesto turns into a thick, pourable consistency; add more water and/or sun-dried tomato oil if the pesto is too thick.

To serve, place a roasted cauliflower steak and a few florets on each plate, top with the sun-dried tomatoes, and spoon the pesto on top. Sprinkle with the Parmesan cheese and serve immediately.

Note: You should be able to get four steaks from a 12-inch-diameter cauliflower head, or two steaks from a 8- or 9-inch head. Even if your steaks fall apart, you can reassemble them on the baking sheet; they will still roast up deliciously. Also, make sure there is enough room for hot air to circulate around the steaks and florets for golden-roasted results; if the sheets seem crowded, remove some cauliflower and roast another time when your oven is on, or add to salads or veggie trays.

Healthy Kitchen Hack: We're always looking for creative and yummy ways to use up the entire veggie, so here are a few more tips to enjoy all parts of that cauliflower or broccoli head. Toss cauliflower or broccoli *leaves* into salads, simmer in soups, or drizzle with olive oil and then roast in a 400°F oven like kale chips. For cauliflower and broccoli *stems*, peel the outer fibrous part of broccoli and slice or dice and then mix into stir-fries, steam with other favorite vegetables, shred into slaws, or pickle them (use our Antipasto Pickles recipe on page 52). Our hands-down favorite Hack is to toss chopped cauliflower stalks and floret "crumbles" into boiling water along with elbow pasta for a mac and cheese upgrade.

Per Serving: Calories: 352; **Total Fat:** 29g; **Saturated Fat:** 4g; **Cholesterol:** 5mg; **Sodium:** 398mg; **Total Carbohydrates:** 20g; **Fiber:** 6g; **Protein:** 10g

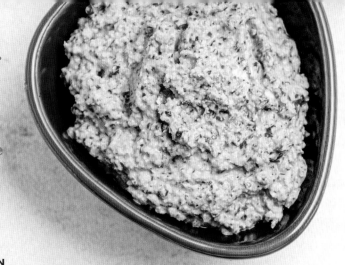

"Toasting the cauliflower steaks on the hot pan worked really well and gave them great flavor. I'll definitely make these again and put the sauce down first to make it like a fancy restaurant meal, it's that good!"

—Pamela from Minneapolis, MN

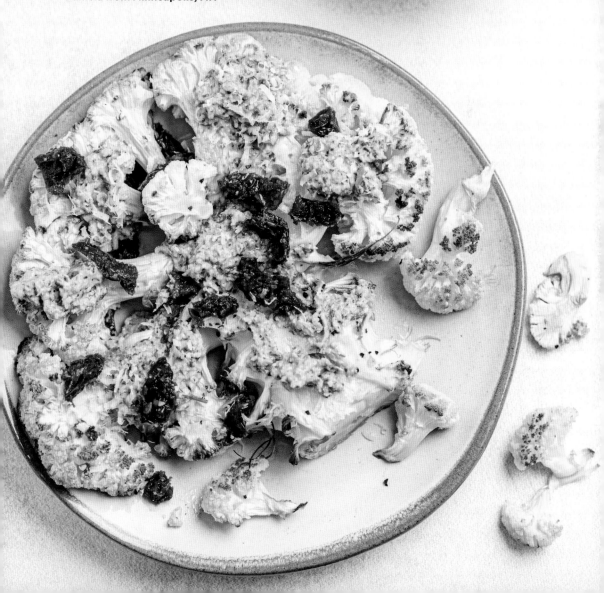

Inside-Out Vegan Cabbage Rolls

SERVES 6
Prep time: 10 minutes
Cook time: 20 minutes

1 small or ½ large head green cabbage (about 6½ cups chopped)

2 tablespoons olive oil

4 scallions (green onions), green and white parts, thinly sliced *Save the stem roots! See page 70*

1 cup uncooked bulgur

¼ teaspoon ground cinnamon

¼ teaspoon ground ginger

¼ teaspoon ground nutmeg

⅛ teaspoon cayenne pepper

2 cups Veggie Scraps Broth (page 120) or low-sodium vegetable broth

1 tablespoon tomato paste

1 (15-ounce) can chickpeas, drained (liquid saved for another use) and rinsed

1 lemon

½ cup chopped walnuts, pistachios, or almonds

½ cup finely chopped fresh mint or basil, leaves and stems

½ teaspoon kosher or sea salt

¼ teaspoon black pepper

Cultures around the globe from North China to Scandinavia boast their signature versions of stuffed cabbage rolls. Mediterranean countries are no different: from Algeria to Lebanon, each recipe features unique aromatic spices and satisfying fillings. This shortcut dish skips the typical double-cooking process of steaming the leaves and then baking the stuffed cabbage. Instead, we just chop up everything and cook it in one pot for all the flavor with none of the fuss. We swap in chickpeas for meat, use bulgur as the grain, and season with a surprising yet tantalizing mix of cinnamon, ginger, and cayenne, which produces layers of sweet, spicy, hot, and savory flavors—not too shabby for a vegan meal!

Cut off the hard cabbage stem at the base (save it in your Veggie Scraps freezer bag—see page 120), then coarsely chop the remaining cabbage, including the outer leaves and inner core. (If using ½ head, see this recipe's Hack.)

Heat the oil in a large stockpot over medium heat. Add the cabbage and scallions and cook, stirring frequently, until the cabbage starts to brown, 4 to 5 minutes. Add the bulgur, cinnamon, ginger, nutmeg, and cayenne and cook, stirring frequently, for 1 minute. Add the broth and tomato paste. Stir together and bring to a boil. Reduce the heat to medium-low, cover, and cook for 5 minutes. Stir well, cover again, and cook for at least an additional 5 minutes or until the cabbage is cooked to your liking. Turn off the heat and stir in the chickpeas. Cover and let sit for another 5 minutes.

Using a Microplane or citrus zester, grate the zest from the lemon into the pot; cut the lemon in half and squeeze in 1 tablespoon juice. (Save the remaining juice for another use.) Add the nuts, herbs, salt, and black pepper and mix well. Serve warm.

Note: If you don't need to keep this recipe vegan and dairy-free, serve each portion with 2 tablespoons plain Greek yogurt on top for stirring into the dish.

Healthy Kitchen Hack: If you have half a head of cabbage from this recipe or another leftover in your fridge, use it to make our Tahini Use-Up-Those-Veggies Slaw (page 75) or toss it into our Very Veggie Sustainable Soup (page 111). Or cut into wedges, brush with olive oil, sprinkle with salt, and roast in the oven at 400°F (if there's room when you already are cooking something else) for about 30 minutes, then serve with your favorite salad dressing or our Zesty Garlic Sauce (page 100).

Per Serving: Calories: 285; Total Fat: 13g; Saturated Fat: 2g; Cholesterol: 0mg; Sodium: 436mg; Total Carbohydrates: 37g; Fiber: 10g; Protein: 10g

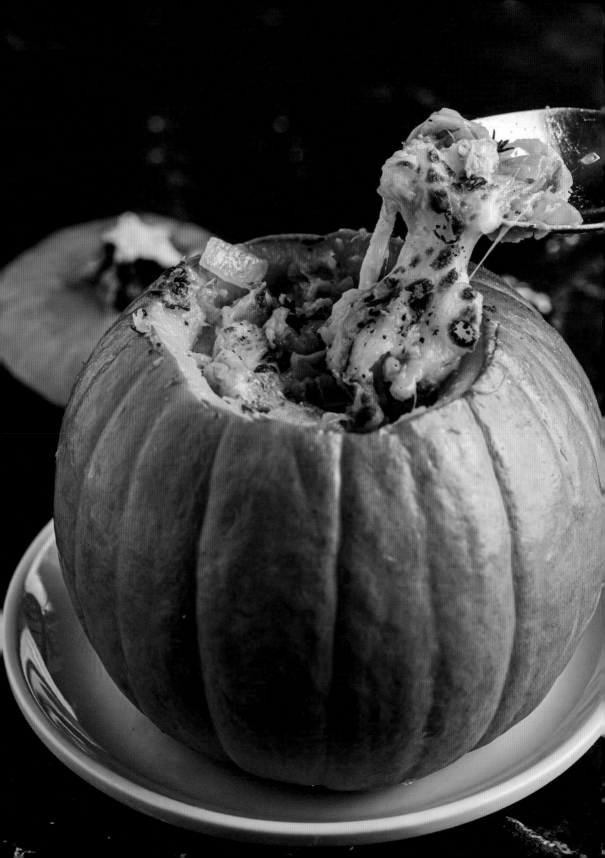

Whole Pumpkin Cheesy Gratin

SERVES 4
Prep time: 15 minutes
Cook time: 30 minutes

1 (3- to 5-pound) sugar or pie pumpkin (make sure it will fit in your microwave)

2 tablespoons extra-virgin olive oil

2 cups chopped onion

1 large apple, cored and chopped

2 thyme sprigs

¼ teaspoon kosher or sea salt

¼ teaspoon black pepper

1 cup Veggie Scraps Broth (page 120) or low-sodium vegetable broth

2 cups cubed crusty whole-grain bread (¾-inch pieces)

1½ cups shredded part-skim mozzarella cheese (about 6 ounces), divided

If you've never cooked a whole pumpkin before, this is the showstopper dish to convince you how easy it can be. For minimal effort, you'll receive maximum accolades (and nutrition!), all packaged in nature's perfect and completely edible vessel. Wow your family and/or guests when you carry this golden stuffed squash to the table, lift the lid, watch the steam rise, and listen to all the oohs and aahs! And then, scoop out the warm gratin with the cheese stretching into long strings. This unforgettable meal is sure to become a seasonal favorite. Serve it up with our Spinach Salad with Balsamic Goat Cheese Dressing (page 84).

Measure or eyeball the size of your pumpkin and arrange the top rack so the top of the pumpkin will be about 4 inches from the heat source. Preheat the broiler to high.

Make several slits around the stem of the pumpkin, in a 5- to 6-inch-diameter circle, to allow steam to release. Microwave the pumpkin (break off the stem if it's too large to fit in the microwave) on high for 6 to 7 minutes, until the flesh is tender enough to cut out but the pumpkin is still firm enough to be used a vessel for the stuffing.

Using oven mitts, transfer the pumpkin to the cutting board to cool slightly, about 5 minutes. Holding the pumpkin with an oven mitt, cut along the steam holes you made and slice off the top to remove the "lid." Set aside for serving. Scoop out the seeds (save them for roasting for another recipe; see page 61). Cut and scrape out most of the flesh from the inside, leaving a ¼- to ½-inch-thick shell. Chop the pumpkin flesh into ¾-inch cubes; you should have about 2 cups.

Heat the oil in a large saucepan or Dutch oven over medium heat. Add the onion and cook, stirring occasionally, until translucent, 5 to 7 minutes. Stir in the pumpkin flesh, apple, thyme, salt, and pepper and cook, stirring occasionally, until the pumpkin starts to turn golden, about 5 minutes. Add the broth and scrape up the browned bits on the bottom. Continue cooking until the pumpkin flesh is tender, 3 to 4 minutes. Add the

continued

bread cubes and 1 cup cheese and cook, stirring, until heated through and the cheese begins to melt. Remove the thyme sprigs and slide in any leaves that have not fallen off the stems.

Transfer the mixture to the pumpkin shell. Top with the remaining ½ cup cheese and broil (without the pumpkin lid) until the cheese is golden brown, 3 to 4 minutes (watch carefully). Remove from the oven.

To serve, replace the lid, bring to the table, and lift the lid when ready to spoon out the gratin.

Healthy Kitchen Hack: This recipe can be stunning with any variety of winter squash—in almost any size—such as acorn, butternut, Hubbard, or spaghetti squash. Some shapes are better suited for cutting the squash in half lengthwise first before scooping out the flesh; just mound the filling on top of both halves before broiling. Serena once served a beautiful 7-pound Cinderella (or calabaza), which is a bright orange, thick-fleshed, squat squash, from her mother-in-law's garden! When the gratin is finished, don't dump the serving vessel. Slice up the pumpkin/squash, microwave until soft, and enjoy the remaining flesh, including the skin, topped with sugar and cinnamon for a snack, or pureed into pumpkin soup; the skin on most pumpkins, especially pie pumpkins, is thin and edible.

Per Serving: Calories: 373; **Total Fat:** 13g; **Saturated Fat:** 5g; **Cholesterol:** 21mg; **Sodium:** 528mg; **Total Carbohydrates:** 51g; **Fiber:** 7g; **Protein:** 15g

"My wife thinks it would be a great showstopping dish for our Thanksgiving dinner. But I want to eat it more often than just on Thanksgiving."

—Kyle from Lakewood, CO

Rustic Roasted Vegetable Crostata

SERVES 6
Prep time: 20 minutes
Cook time: 25 minutes

½ batch Speedy Pizza Dough recipe (page 138), at room temperature, *or* 1 pound store-bought pizza dough

8 ounces broccolini

1 small yellow squash or zucchini

½ batch Romesco Sauce (page 91) *or* 1½ cups your favorite tomato sauce, divided

3 teaspoons extra-virgin olive oil, divided

¼ teaspoon kosher or sea salt

¼ teaspoon black pepper

1 (14-ounce) can quartered artichokes (not marinated), drained (liquid saved for another use)

1 (2.25-ounce) can sliced black olives (about ½ cup), drained (liquid saved for another use)

2 ounces Manchego cheese

2 teaspoons fresh thyme leaves

Not quite a pizza or a pie, this savory free-form tart is straightforward and bursting with color and seasonal goodness. Here we feature late summer veggies, but feel free to swap in your fresh favorites during their peak of ripeness: try asparagus, leeks, and arugula in spring, tomatoes and onions in early summer, and in cooler months, mushrooms, cauliflower, and broccoli. And of course, canned or jarred ingredients like artichokes, olives, mushrooms, tomatoes, roasted peppers, corn, and capers give you endless year-round topping options.

Preheat the oven to 425°F. Line a large rimmed baking sheet with parchment paper.

Using a rolling pin dusted with flour, roll the pizza dough into a 15-inch circle and place it on the lined baking sheet. Set aside.

Using a vegetable peeler, remove the outer skin of the broccolini stalks (compost or store in freezer bag to make our Veggie Scraps Broth on page 120). For any thick stalks, cut in half lengthwise, then cut all the broccolini into 1-inch pieces. Cut the squash in half lengthwise and in half again lengthwise so you have four long pieces, then cut into ¼-inch-thick slices.

In a medium bowl, mix together the chopped broccolini (including any leaves) and squash with about ½ cup Romesco sauce, 2 teaspoons oil, salt, and pepper until all the vegetables are coated.

Spoon about ¼ cup of the remaining Romesco sauce into the center of the dough circle. With the back of the spoon, spread the sauce to within 2 inches of the edge. Add the broccolini and squash mixture and spread out to within 2 inches of the edge. Scatter the artichoke hearts and black olives all over. Drizzle the remaining ¾ cup Romesco sauce over the vegetables. Using a vegetable peeler, shave pieces of the Manchego cheese over the top, then sprinkle with thyme. Fold about 1½ inches of the edges of the dough up and over some of the vegetables, leaving most of the toppings

continued

exposed in the center. Brush the folded-over crust with the remaining 1 teaspoon oil.

Bake for about 25 minutes or until the edges and bottom of the crust are golden brown. Let cool for 10 minutes on a wire rack, then cut into 6 pieces and serve.

Healthy Kitchen Hack: Turn this savory crostata sweet! Instead of the vegetables, Romesco sauce, and cheese, mix up a batch of our Ugly Fruit Jam (page 259), then add 1 cup finely chopped fruit you have on hand. Spoon into the center of the dough and follow the same instructions for folding over the dough and baking. If desired, before serving, sprinkle with the thyme leaves or other fresh herbs, like mint or basil, and some fresh lemon zest.

Per Serving: Calories: 281; Total Fat: 10g; Saturated Fat: 3g; Cholesterol: 11mg; Sodium: 620mg; Total Carbohydrates: 37g; Fiber: 5g; Protein: 18g

"Since broccolini and Manchego are new to me, I wasn't sure I'd like the taste, but I did! I had some extra veggie filling, which I baked in a small dish with extra sauce and cheese alongside the crostata."

—Elise from Kensington, MD

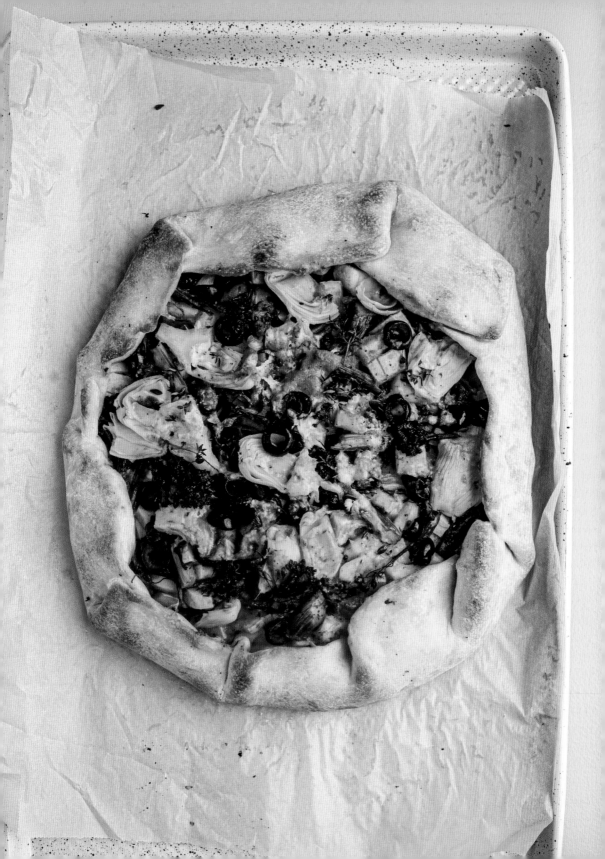

"Not Quite Paella" Farro Medley

SERVES 6
Prep time: 10 minutes
Cook time: 30 minutes

Paella is one of the most iconic Spanish dishes. Traditionally, it is studded with chicken and seafood; we instead stirred up an enticingly turmeric-colored vegetable medley featuring chewy, fiber-rich farro. (Although if you love little fishes, feel free to add a few tins of smoked seafood!) And in another tinkering with tradition, Deanna tried replacing the chicken broth with the flavorful liquids from the recipe's canned and jarred vegetables and was excited that it totally worked (yay for using *everything* from those canned veggies!). As we suggest in almost every recipe, feel free to swap in even more ingredients you have on hand (see ideas in the Hack).

½ (1-pound) bag frozen baby lima beans

1 tablespoon extra-virgin olive oil

8 ounces mushrooms (any type), chopped

1 cup chopped celery stalks and leaves

1 medium onion (any type), chopped

2 garlic cloves, minced

1½ cups uncooked pearled or 10-minute farro

¾ teaspoon smoked paprika

¾ teaspoon ground turmeric

1 tablespoon tomato paste

1 (14.5-ounce) can diced tomatoes, drained and liquid reserved

1 (14-ounce) can artichokes hearts, drained, quartered, and liquid reserved

1 (12-ounce) jar roasted red peppers, drained, sliced, and liquid reserved

1 (2.25-ounces) can sliced black olives, drained and liquid reserved

1 bay leaf

¼ teaspoon kosher or sea salt

¼ teaspoon black pepper

¼ cup chopped fresh parsley or cilantro, leaves and stems

1 lemon, cut into wedges

Pour the lima beans into a small bowl and let them sit on the counter to thaw while you start cooking.

Heat the oil in a large skillet over medium heat. Add the mushrooms, celery, and onion and cook, stirring occasionally, for 5 minutes or until the mushrooms just start to wilt. Add the garlic and cook for 1 minute, stirring frequently. Add the farro, smoked paprika, and turmeric and cook for 1 minute, stirring frequently. Add the tomato paste and cook, stirring frequently, for 1 minute or until fragrant.

Pour the liquid from the tomatoes, artichokes, red peppers, and olives into a large measuring cup. Add 2 cups of the liquid to the skillet, along with the bay leaf. Bring to a simmer, reduce the heat to medium-low, and cook, without stirring, for about 15 minutes or until there is barely any liquid left on the bottom of the pan. Turn off the heat. On top of the farro, spread out the lima beans, tomatoes, artichokes, red peppers, olives, salt, and pepper. Gently stir (just a few stirs) the vegetables into the top layer of the farro. Let sit for 10 minutes, then remove the bay leaf. Sprinkle with the parsley or cilantro and serve right out of the skillet, with lemon wedges for squeezing.

Healthy Kitchen Hack: Make this dish different every time with a variety of frozen, fresh, and/or canned veggies. The combinations are endless!

- *Frozen veggie options:* peas, broccoli, green beans, corn, edamame, spinach
- *Fresh veggie options:* carrots, hot peppers, broccoli, spinach, cabbage
- *Canned veggie options:* corn, chickpeas, potatoes, mushrooms

---

Per Serving: Calories: 331; Total Fat: 5g; Saturated Fat: 1g; Cholesterol: 0mg; Sodium: 449mg; Total Carbohydrates: 63g; Fiber: 13g; Protein: 14g

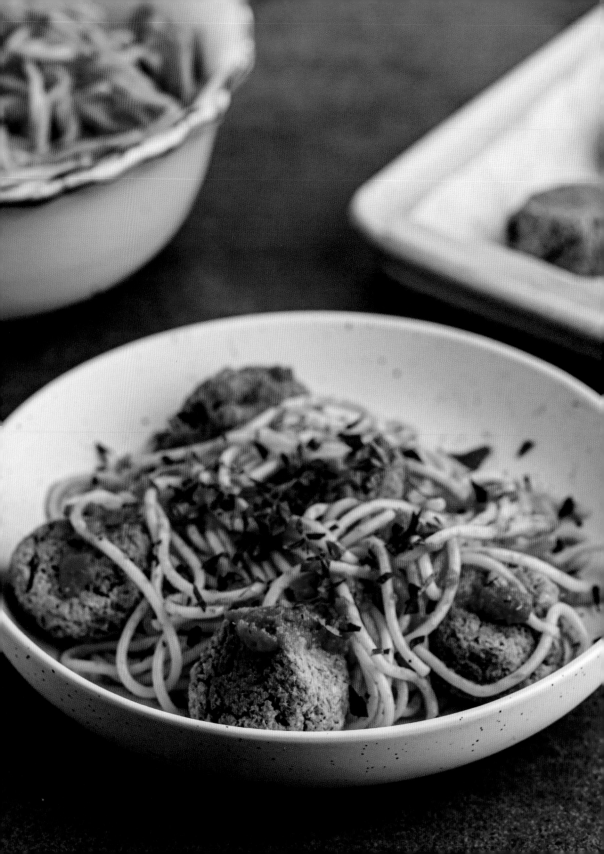

Ricotta and Lentil "Meat" Balls with Marinara

SERVES 6
Prep time: 15 minutes
Cook time: 25 minutes

2½ cups cooked lentils (see page 170) *or* drained canned lentils

⅓ cup fresh parsley, leaves and stems, plus more for garnish if desired

4 garlic cloves, peeled

1 batch Made-in-Minutes Homemade Ricotta Cheese (page 48) **plus** 1 tablespoon whey *or* ¾ cup store-bought whole-milk ricotta cheese

½ cup panko bread crumbs

¼ cup grated Parmesan or Pecorino Romano cheese

2 teaspoons dried oregano

1 large egg

½ teaspoon kosher or sea salt, divided

½ teaspoon black pepper, divided

1 tablespoon extra-virgin olive oil

1 (28-ounce) can crushed tomatoes

1 teaspoon balsamic vinegar

1 teaspoon honey

Deanna was a bit skeptical that an iconic Italian-style meatball could be made without meat, but creating this recipe changed her mind. Lentils—rather amazing little plants in terms of nutrient density, cooking versatility, and crop sustainability—work well as a ground beef extender or substitute. When they're paired with typical meatball ingredients like parsley, garlic, and ricotta, the results are pretty spot-on. Serve up these "meat" balls in classic style with spaghetti or in rolls or pita pockets for sandwiches.

Arrange the oven racks to the upper-middle and lower-middle positions. Preheat the oven to 400°F. Line two large rimmed baking sheets with parchment paper.

In a food processor or high-powered blender, puree the lentils, parsley, and garlic until a thick puree forms, then transfer to a large mixing bowl. Add the ricotta cheese, panko, grated cheese, oregano, egg, and ¼ teaspoon each salt and pepper. Using your hands, gently mix the ingredients together. Using a 1½-tablespoon scoop or measuring spoon, shape the mixture into 1¼-inch balls (you should end up with about 35 lentil-balls) and place them on the prepared baking sheets.

Brush the tops of the lentil-balls with the oil. Bake for 12 minutes, then remove the sheets from the oven. Working quickly, use a spoon to turn over each lentil-ball, then return the sheets to the oven on the opposite racks. Bake for another 10 to 12 minutes, or until the lentil-balls are slightly golden brown in spots on both sides.

When the lentil-balls are nearly done, pour the crushed tomatoes into a medium saucepan over medium heat. Mix in the vinegar, honey, and remaining ¼ teaspoon each salt and pepper and bring to a low simmer.

Serve the lentil-balls immediately by portioning them into bowls and spooning the marinara sauce over them (avoid adding all the lentil-balls to the pot of sauce

continued

as they break down easily—see the Hack). Sprinkle with additional chopped parsley if desired. Let any leftover lentil-balls cool completely, then transfer to a freezer-safe container and store in the freezer for up to 3 months.

Flavor Options

Use this recipe as a template to explore new Mediterranean-flavored lentil-ball variations:

Greek: Add ½ teaspoon dried dill and ½ cup finely chopped olives, and replace the ricotta with crumbled feta.

Moroccan: Add ½ cup finely chopped raisins and replace the oregano with 1 teaspoon ground cumin and ½ teaspoon ground cinnamon.

Spanish: Add ½ cup diced roasted red peppers and replace 1 teaspoon of the oregano with ½ teaspoon smoked paprika and ½ teaspoon dried thyme.

Middle Eastern: Add the grated zest of 1 lemon and replace 1 teaspoon of the oregano with 1 teaspoon za'atar.

Healthy Kitchen Hack: We recommend spooning the marinara sauce over the lentil-balls (and spaghetti if desired) rather than simmering them in the sauce because they're fragile and may break apart. But as Deanna discovered when she was testing this recipe and stirred her sauce a little too eagerly, broken lentil-balls make for an *excellent* vegetarian Bolognese sauce! Simply crumble and stir about 10 of the cooked lentil-balls into the marinara as it simmers and serve with your favorite cooked pasta.

Per Serving: Calories: 276; Total Fat: 7g; Saturated Fat: 4g; Cholesterol: 50mg; Sodium: 537mg; Total Carbohydrates: 40g; Fiber: 7g; Protein: 17g

Mascarpone Egg Scramble with Carrot "Bacon" Bits

SERVES 6
Prep time: 10 minutes
Cook time: 10 minutes

1 pound carrots, unpeeled and diced

2½ tablespoons extra-virgin olive oil, divided

1 tablespoon less-sodium soy sauce

2 teaspoons honey

½ teaspoon kosher or sea salt, divided

½ teaspoon black pepper, divided

¼ teaspoon ground cumin

¼ teaspoon garlic powder

¼ teaspoon smoked paprika

8 large eggs

2 tablespoons chopped fresh chives, divided

1 tablespoon 2% milk

½ cup mascarpone cheese

Toasted bread or pita bread, for serving (optional)

Making breakfast food for dinner is a familiar meal strategy in both Serena's and Deanna's households. Growing up, Deanna loved when her mom served scrambled eggs mixed with chopped bacon for dinner. It felt like a special meal. Now as a mother, she realizes it was a quick-fix, "Mom needs to whip up something super fast" kind of dinner. But this 20-minute recipe is a definite upgrade to your classic breakfast eggs with the addition of luxurious, ultra-smooth mascarpone cheese and surprisingly umami-rich, smoky charred carrot bits. Whenever you see carrots with the tops at the store or farmers' market, grab them! They tend to be super sweet *and* you can take advantage of those tasty "bonus" greens to make our vibrant Carrot Top Pesto (page 148).

Arrange the top oven rack about 4 inches under the broiler. Preheat the broiler to high 5 minutes before using. Coat a large rimmed baking sheet with cooking spray.

In a medium bowl, combine the carrots, 1½ tablespoons oil, soy sauce, honey, ¼ teaspoon each salt and pepper, cumin, garlic powder, and smoked paprika. Toss until the carrots are well coated. Spread out on the prepared sheet. Broil the carrots for 4 minutes and then stir. Broil for an additional 2 to 4 minutes or until the carrots just start to blacken. Set aside.

Meanwhile, wipe out the bowl and whisk the eggs, 1 tablespoon chives, milk, and remaining ¼ teaspoon each salt and pepper until frothy.

Heat the remaining 1 tablespoon oil in a large skillet over medium-low heat. Add the egg mixture and cook, undisturbed, for 1 minute, then cook, stirring occasionally with a spatula, for 2 minutes. Spoon in the mascarpone and gently fold into the eggs until there are pockets of mascarpone distributed throughout the eggs. Cook, stirring occasionally to fold the cooked eggs from the outside into the rest of the mixture, until the eggs are soft scrambled, another 3 to 5 minutes. Remove from the heat.

continued

Mascarpone Egg Scramble with Carrot "Bacon" Bits *(continued)*

Serve the eggs alongside the roasted carrot bits (or mix the carrots into the pan with eggs) and sprinkle with the remaining 1 tablespoon chives. Serve with toasted bread or pita if you like.

Healthy Kitchen Hack: Yes, you *can* reheat scrambled eggs to be as light and fluffy as they are when they are first cooked! So, make a double batch, refrigerate, and when it's time to eat, reheat them in either of the following ways:

- Heat a teaspoon or two of olive oil in a skillet over medium heat. Add the eggs and cook, stirring frequently, until warm, 1 to 3 minutes **OR**

- Put the eggs in a microwave-safe bowl, partially cover with a plate, and microwave for 15 seconds. Remove, pour out any liquid, stir, and reheat for another 15 seconds or until the eggs are warm.

Per Serving: Calories: 349; Total Fat: 29g; Saturated Fat: 14g; Cholesterol: 295mg; Sodium: 401mg; Total Carbohydrates: 12g; Fiber: 2g; Protein: 11g

Roasted Thyme Mushrooms over Parmesan Polenta Squares

SERVES 6
Prep time: 10 minutes
Cook time: 40 minutes

8 tablespoons grated Parmesan or Pecorino cheese, divided

2 cups 2% milk

½ teaspoon kosher or sea salt, divided

1 cup yellow cornmeal

2 pounds mushrooms (any type), coarsely chopped

¼ cup extra-virgin olive oil

3 tablespoons tomato paste

2 garlic cloves, minced

2 teaspoons red wine vinegar or balsamic vinegar

2 teaspoons dried thyme

¼ teaspoon black pepper

¼ cup fresh parsley or cilantro, leaves and stems, finely chopped

This one's dedicated to all our mushroom lovers (including Deanna's cat Pete, who eats them with his paw). Besides being one of the most sustainable veggies around (mushrooms can grow almost anywhere in a small amount of space), they are also super abundant, with more than 2,000 edible varieties! So, get out of your white button mushroom rut and try those creminis, shiitakes, portobellos, oysters, or any other mushrooms on your next trip to the store or the farmers' market (or the forest, if you're the foraging type!). Then use them for these plant-rich, soul-satisfying polenta bites. (Check out Serena's Healthy Kitchen Hack on page 163 for more mushroom options.)

Arrange the oven racks to the upper-middle and lower-middle positions. Preheat the oven to 425°F. Line a 9 × 13-inch rimmed baking sheet or baking dish with parchment paper or coat with cooking spray. Sprinkle with 2 tablespoons grated cheese.

Pour the milk and 1½ cups water into a medium stockpot. Add ¼ teaspoon salt and bring to a boil over medium-high heat (do not let the liquid boil over). Reduce the heat to medium and slowly pour in the cornmeal, whisking constantly for about 1 minute. Reduce the heat to medium-low and continue to cook, whisking frequently, until the polenta is thickened and smooth, 6 to 8 minutes. Remove from the heat and mix in ¼ cup grated cheese. Immediately pour the polenta over the cheese on the prepared baking sheet. Using a spatula, evenly spread and smooth out the polenta mixture. Sprinkle with the remaining 2 tablespoons grated cheese.

While the polenta cooks on the stove, spread out the mushrooms on a large rimmed baking sheet. (It's fine if they seem crowded as they will shrink during cooking.) In a small bowl, whisk together the oil, tomato paste, garlic, vinegar, thyme, pepper, and remaining ¼ teaspoon

continued

salt (this mixture will be thick). Spoon over the mushrooms (reserve the bowl for later use) and stir or toss with your hands until all the mushrooms are lightly coated.

Transfer the polenta sheet to the upper rack and the mushroom sheet to the lower rack in the oven. Bake for 15 minutes. Remove the mushrooms from the oven and carefully tilt the sheet into the reserved bowl to pour off most of the juices, leaving the mushrooms on the sheet. Stir the mushrooms and spread them out again. Move the polenta to the bottom rack and place the mushrooms on the upper rack. Bake for an additional 10 minutes. If the polenta is golden brown on the edges and in some areas on the top, remove from the oven; otherwise, bake for another 2 to 5 minutes. At this time, stir the mushrooms and bake for another 5 minutes, until they are dark brown and reduced in size. Remove from the oven.

Let cool for at least 5 minutes, then cut the polenta squares into thirds lengthwise and sixths crosswise to make 18 portions. To serve, place 3 polenta squares on each plate, top with one-sixth of the mushrooms, and drizzle with some of the reserved mushroom juices. Sprinkle each plate with 2 teaspoons herbs and serve warm.

Healthy Kitchen Hack: To reheat leftover polenta squares (if there are any left!), toast them in a toaster oven, reheat in a skillet on the stove, or zap under the broiler. Serve as breakfast with scrambled eggs, or spread your favorite tomato/pizza sauce on top of a few squares to enjoy as a quick snack. Or cut them into cubes, toast, and toss into soups or over salads (think croutons!).

Per Serving: Calories: 281; Total Fat: 14g; Saturated Fat: 4g; Cholesterol: 14mg; Sodium: 672mg; Total Carbohydrates: 30g; Fiber: 4g; Protein: 12g

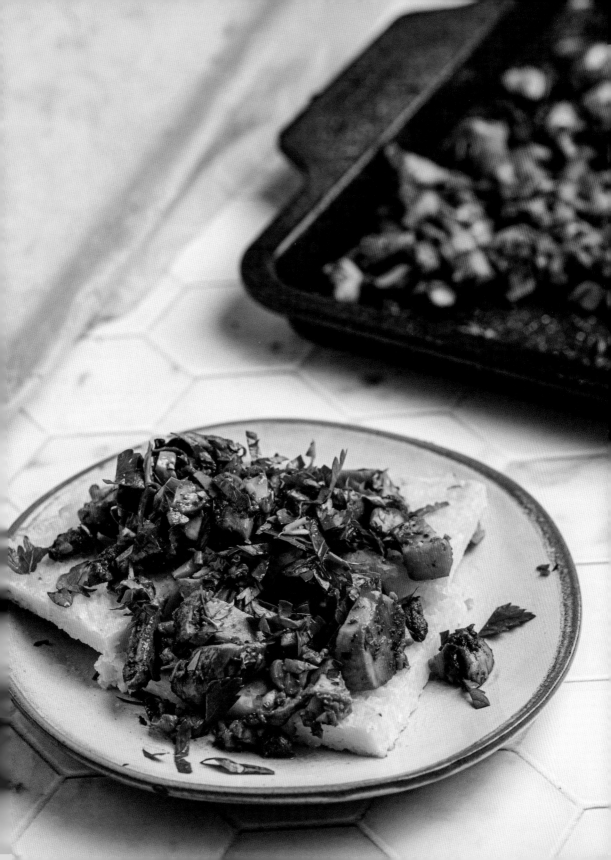

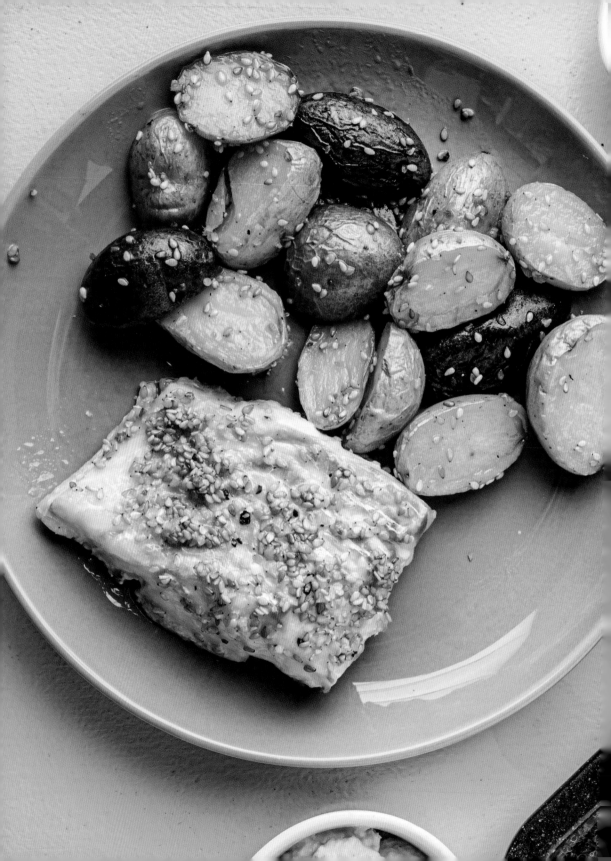

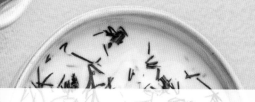

Seafood

Microwaved White Fish with Tomatoes and Chives

SERVES 4
Prep time: 10 minutes
Cook time: 5 minutes

1 lemon

4 tablespoons chopped fresh chives, divided

2 teaspoons extra-virgin olive oil

4 (4-ounce) frozen skin-on or skinless white fish fillets (from the More Sustainable Seafood Choices List on page 19), thawed

¼ teaspoon kosher or sea salt

¼ teaspoon black pepper

½ cup chopped fresh tomatoes or canned (undrained) diced tomatoes

Tap into some microwave magic for perfectly cooked fish. We've included a version of this fish cooking method in each of our cookbooks because it was such a revelation the first time we tried it—and now we make it almost weekly this way. Topped with bright red tomatoes and fresh green chives, this fish dish will look appetizing any time of year, especially when you need dinner in a hurry. Choose your favorite eco-friendly frozen white fish (see our list on page 19); if you didn't remember to thaw your fish overnight in the fridge, see our quick thaw methods on page 206.

Using a Microplane or citrus zester, grate the zest from the lemon into a glass pie dish or large microwave-safe bowl, then cut the lemon in half and squeeze in 2 tablespoons lemon juice. (Save the remaining juice for another use.) Add 2 tablespoons chives and the oil, then whisk.

Pat the fillets dry and season both sides with the salt and pepper. Transfer the fillets to the lemon oil mixture and flip a few times until the fillets are fully coated. With the fillets skin-side down (if they have skin), fold each fillet in half crosswise so that all fillets fit inside the dish. Cover the dish with a microwave-safe plate, leaving a small gap at the edge to vent the steam.

Microwave on high for 3 minutes. Carefully remove the hot dish with oven mitts and let some of the steam escape before removing the plate. Check the fillets with a fork to see if the fish is just starting to separate into flakes. If any part doesn't look cooked, cover again as before and microwave in 20-second increments until done.

Transfer the cooked fish to a serving platter. Top with the remaining 2 tablespoons chives and the tomatoes. Pour the sauce from the bottom of the glass dish over the top.

Healthy Kitchen Hack: Once you try this microwave fish method, we think you may love it enough to make it weekly as we do! Here, in no particular order, are our *Top 10 Fish Toppers* for some variety:

1) Carrot Top Pesto (page 148)
2) Honey, Orange, and Scallion Vinaigrette (page 70)
3) Romesco Sauce (page 91)
4) Mint Cucumber Salad (page 80)
5) Zesty Garlic Sauce (page 100)
6) Orange slices with honey: top before microwaving
7) Everything bagel seasoning: top before microwaving
8) Minced garlic and crushed red pepper: top before microwaving
9) Chopped olives and za'atar spice: top before microwaving
10) Chopped Antipasto Pickles (page 52): top before serving

Per Serving: Calories: 111; Total Fat: 4g; Saturated Fat: 1g; Cholesterol: 61mg; Sodium: 212mg; Total Carbohydrates: 2g; Fiber: 1g; Protein: 17g

So-Good Grilled Fish on Limes

SERVES 4
Prep time: 15 minutes
Cook time: 10 minutes

1 pound frozen, skin-on or skinless white or fatty fish fillet(s) (from the More Sustainable Seafood Choices List on page 19), thawed

3 large or 4 medium limes

1 tablespoon extra-virgin olive oil

¼ teaspoon garlic powder

¼ teaspoon kosher or sea salt

¼ teaspoon black pepper

"What a great summer meal! We loved how the grilled flavor was light and we could even taste the citrus just from the fish cooking on limes."

—Jim and Leah from Halifax, PA

Serena didn't always like the intense heat of the grill (since food can go from raw to burnt in minutes!), but then she read about grilling fish on lemons and limes to create smoky, citrus-infused seafood, and she was in. Her first attempt resulted in perfectly cooked fish that didn't stick to the grill, along with lightly charred lime slices to squeeze over the fillets. Serve this with our Tahini Use-Up-Those-Veggies Slaw (page 75).

Pat the fish dry and let it sit for 10 minutes. Meanwhile, coat the cold grill grate with cooking spray, then preheat the grill to 400°F, or medium-high heat.

Cut the limes into ¼-inch slices (you should have at least 4 middle slices plus 6 to 10 end slices, depending on how many limes you start with). Squeeze the end lime slices into a small bowl until you have 1 tablespoon juice, then save those ends to clean the grill (see the Hack following this recipe). Add the oil and garlic powder to the lime juice and whisk to combine.

Brush both sides of the fish with the lime juice mixture and sprinkle evenly with salt and pepper.

Using tongs, carefully arrange the middle lime slices on the grill in the size and shape of the fish fillet(s). Lay the fillet(s) directly on top of the lime slices (skin-side down if your fish has skin). Close the lid and grill until the fish is just opaque, about 10 minutes for 1-inch-thick fillets, 8 minutes for ¾-inch fillets, and 5 minutes for ½-inch fillets. Using a wide metal spatula, carefully transfer the fish to a platter, then remove the charred limes to serve with the fish.

Healthy Kitchen Hack: Our favorite no-mess trick to clean your grill recycles leftover citrus! After the grill cools completely, rub the grates with used lemon or lime halves or ends (the natural citric acid helps remove build-up). Crumple up a piece of (preferably recycled!) aluminum foil and scrub until all the residue is removed. Remove the grill grate and rinse off with a garden hose.

Per Serving: Calories: 186; Total Fat: 11g; Saturated Fat: 3.3g; Cholesterol: 70mg; Sodium: 120mg; Total Carbohydrates: 2g; Fiber: 0g; Protein: 21g

Barley, Corn, and Mackerel Medley

SERVES 4
Prep time: 10 minutes
Cook time: 15 minutes

1⅓ cups quick pearl barley (see Note)

1⅓ cups frozen corn kernels

1 lemon

2 tablespoons extra-virgin olive oil

1 garlic clove, minced

½ teaspoon black pepper

¼ teaspoon crushed red pepper

¼ teaspoon kosher or sea salt

2 (4- to 6-ounce) tins boneless, skinless mackerel in oil, drained

1 bell pepper (any color), seeded and chopped

1 cup chopped fresh cilantro or parsley, leaves and stems

Admittedly, there were some confused looks on Serena's guests' faces when she announced that she was serving barley with corn and mackerel for lunch. We get it—mackerel isn't in most people's recipe repertoire. But her friends ended up loving this dish and one commented how mackerel was like a smoother, luxurious-tasting canned tuna. We hope this recipe encourages you to purchase some mackerel to celebrate this small, sustainable fish that's rich in healthy omega-3 fats as well as a tasty option for any canned tuna recipe (see this recipe's Healthy Kitchen Hack).

Cook the barley according to the package instructions, without salt. Transfer to a colander and stir in the frozen corn to cool the barley and thaw the corn. Set aside over a bowl and continue to cool.

Using a Microplane or citrus zester, grate the zest from the lemon over a large serving bowl, then cut the lemon in half and squeeze in 2 tablespoons juice. (Save any remaining lemon juice for another use.) Add the oil, garlic, black pepper, crushed red pepper, and salt and whisk to combine. Add the barley-corn mixture along with the mackerel, bell pepper, and cilantro and stir to combine. Serve right away, or store in a covered container in the refrigerator to serve later—you can eat it warm, at room temperature, or chilled!

Note: We used "quick" barley, which cooks in 10 minutes and for which 1 serving is ⅓ cup. If you have a different pearl barley, make enough for 4 servings and adjust the cooking time per the package instructions.

Healthy Kitchen Hack: During our recipe testing for this book, we both have had conversations with the cashiers at our local grocery stores about the rising popularity of canned seafood, including mackerel in oil, which is hands-down Serena's favorite. Swap it for canned tuna in tuna sandwiches, tuna noodle casserole, or tuna burgers.

Per Serving (using 4-ounce cans mackerel): **Calories: 450; Total Fat: 22g; Saturated Fat: 4g; Cholesterol: 20mg; Sodium: 337mg; Total Carbohydrates: 51g; Fiber: 8g; Protein: 15g**

Oven Roasted Whole Fish

SERVES 4
Prep time: 15 minutes
Cook time: 20 minutes

1 (2- to 3-pound) whole fish, cleaned and scaled

½ teaspoon kosher or sea salt, divided

½ teaspoon black pepper, divided

1 small onion (any type), thinly sliced

2 lemons, 1 thinly sliced and 1 cut into wedges

2 tablespoons extra-virgin olive oil, divided

3–4 thyme sprigs *or* 2 rosemary sprigs

¼ teaspoon crushed red pepper (optional)

This might be one of the most rewarding recipes in this book. The wow-factor of presenting a whole fish to the table is on par with the Thanksgiving turkey, but a whole fish is much easier to prepare and quicker to cook. And it's the Mediterranean way, as each country surrounding the sea has its local favorite fish, often prepared simply as we do here with olive oil, lemons, and local wild herbs. But we get it, prepping a whole fish can be intimidating. So start by visiting the fish counter at your local grocery store and checking out the whole fish on display. They come cleaned (insides removed) and scaled, but the head is usually still on (which is great for fish stock; see the Hack after this recipe). That cleaned cavity is perfect to stuff with aromatics, much like a whole turkey. As for which type of fish to buy, ask the fishmonger what is local or check our suggested list on page 19. Or perhaps, you're lucky enough to know someone who likes to fish who will share their bounty!

Preheat the oven to 400°F. Coat a large rimmed baking sheet with cooking spray.

Place the fish on the prepared baking sheet. Sprinkle the inside of the cavity with ¼ teaspoon each salt and black pepper. Lay in a layer of onion slices and then a layer of lemon slices; drizzle with 1 tablespoon oil. Add the thyme or rosemary and sprinkle with the crushed red pepper (if using). Close the fish cavity. Drizzle the remaining 1 tablespoon oil all over the outside of the fish and sprinkle with the remaining ¼ teaspoon each salt and black pepper.

Roast for about 20 minutes or until the flesh at the thickest part is just beginning to flake.

Right before serving, remove the cooked lemons and onions and arrange on the sides of the baking sheet, then bring the whole baking sheet to the table. Using a fork, gently lift out pieces of fish from under the skin, serving each with cooked lemons and onions if desired. Serve with the lemon wedges on the side. Compost the remaining skin but save the bones (including the head) for stock (see the Hack).

Healthy Kitchen Hack: Don't toss the fish head and bones! Store them in a freezer container and save them to make fish stock. In a Dutch oven or large pot, heat 2 tablespoons olive oil. Add 3 to 4 cups total chopped onions, carrots, and celery and cook until soft but not brown. Add 2 bay leaves, 2 teaspoons dried thyme, ¾ teaspoon salt, and the leftover fish head and bones (as well as any mussel shells or other frozen saved seafood scraps). Pour in 1 to 2 cups dry white wine, vegetable broth, or water, then add more water to cover everything. Simmer over medium heat for 45 minutes (but do not boil and do not cook for longer to avoid bitter broth). Strain through a fine-mesh strainer (except the very bottom sediment—leave that in the pot). Compost the strained fish bones and sediment. Enjoy the broth plain or as the base for our Smoked Seafood Farro "Risotto" (page 218) or Any-Day Bouillabaisse (page 119).

Per Serving: **Calories: 209; Total Fat: 12g; Saturated Fat: 2g; Cholesterol: 51mg; Sodium: 285mg; Total Carbohydrates: 10g; Fiber: 1g; Protein: 17g**

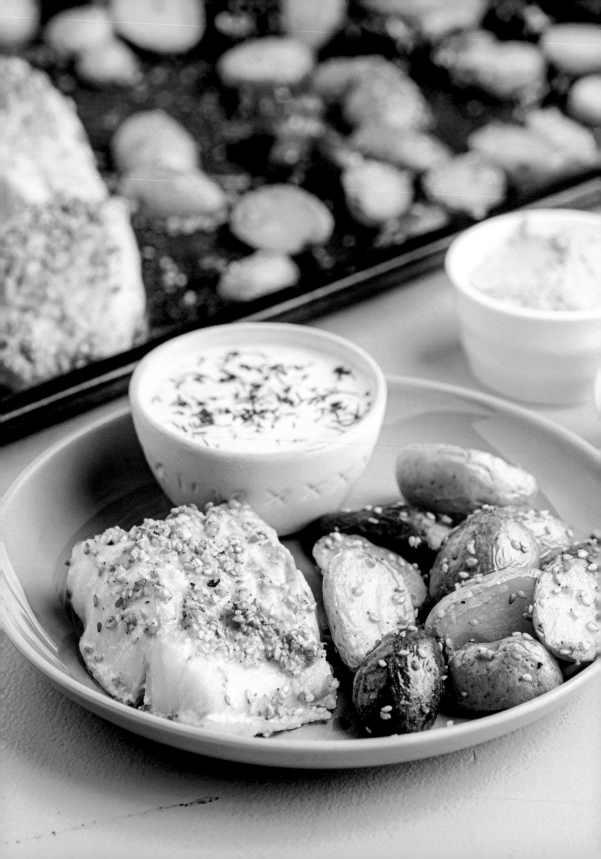

Sheet Pan Sesame Seed Fish with Baby Potatoes

SERVES 4
Prep time: 15 minutes
Cook time: 20 minutes

3 tablespoons sesame seeds

2 garlic cloves, minced, *or* 2 teaspoons dried minced garlic, *or* ¼ teaspoon garlic powder

½ teaspoon black pepper

¼ teaspoon kosher or sea salt

1 pound baby potatoes, sliced ¼ inch thick

3 tablespoons extra-virgin olive oil, divided

4 (4-ounce) frozen skinless white fish fillets (from the More Sustainable Seafood Choices on page 19), thawed

"TARTAR" SAUCE

¾ cup plain 2% Greek yogurt

½ cup finely chopped Antipasto Pickles (page 52) plus ¼ cup pickle liquid *or* store-bought sweet-and-sour-style pickles and liquid

1 tablespoon finely chopped fresh dill *or* 1 teaspoon dried dill, plus more for garnish

1 teaspoon honey (optional)

We like to think of this dish as our oven-baked Mediterranean version of fish and chips. It's inspired by Deanna's obsession with everything bagel seasoning, a mixture brimming with toasted sesame seeds and garlic. Those humble seeds become the star of the show in this fish dish, as they pack so much flavor and texture—not to mention fiber, calcium, and plant protein—into their tiny size. Serve with our speedy, creamy tartar-style sauce or (double) dip your fish and potatoes into our Silky-Smooth Black Pepper and Za'atar Eggplant Dip (page 58), Romesco Sauce (page 91), or Lemon Hummus (page 231). Or if you're feeling ambitious, serve with an array of all the dippers!

Preheat the oven to 425°F. Coat a large rimmed baking sheet with cooking spray.

In a large bowl, mix the sesame seeds, garlic, pepper, and salt. Remove 1 tablespoon of the spice mix and set aside. Add the potatoes and 2 tablespoons olive oil to the large bowl and toss well until the potatoes are completely covered. Spread the potatoes out on the prepared baking sheet and bake for 10 minutes.

While the potatoes bake, pat the fillets dry and transfer to a plate. If one side of a fillet is thicker than the other, fold the thinner piece under so the fillet is more uniform in thickness. In the same large bowl you used for the potatoes, whisk together the reserved 1 tablespoon spice mix and remaining 1 tablespoon oil. Spoon the mixture over the fish and spread it evenly over the top of each piece.

Remove the baking sheet from the oven. Stir the potatoes and push them to the side to free up about one-third of the space for the fish fillets. Transfer the fish to the open area of the sheet and return it to the

continued

Sheet Pan Sesame Seed Fish with Baby Potatoes *(continued)*

oven. Bake for 8 to 10 minutes, until the potatoes are slightly crisp on the edges and the fish just starts to flake (for fillets that are less than 1 inch thick, bake for about 6 minutes and then check for doneness).

Meanwhile, make the "tartar" sauce. In a small bowl, whisk together the yogurt, finely chopped pickles, pickle juice, and dill. If your pickle juice does not contain sugar or you don't have any carrots or sweet pepper pickles, you may want to whisk in the optional honey to cut the acidity. If you like, garnish the sauce with more dill.

Serve the fish and potatoes warm along with the "tartar" sauce.

Healthy Kitchen Hack: As much as we love the convenience and sustainability of frozen seafood, we sometimes find the final hurdle to cooking it is remembering to defrost it. While the safety gold standard for thawing fish and shellfish is doing it slowly (overnight or up to 24 hours in the refrigerator in a container), we have some shortcuts. Submerge the sealed bag of seafood in a bowl of cool (not ice-cold) water and transfer to the refrigerator. Check on it every 30 minutes or so, replacing the now-cold water with cool water, until the fish is thawed. Depending on the thickness of your fish, this method can shave several hours off the overnight thaw method. Or, you can cook some seafood straight from the freezer in the oven if you aren't flavoring it. First, separate any pieces that stick together. Transfer to a wire rack with a large rimmed baking sheet underneath to catch the excess water from the melting ice in the oven and add a few more minutes to the cooking time. Once you defrost your seafood, be sure to cook it within a few days and resist the urge to refreeze as this will affect the taste and texture.

Per Serving: Calories: 285; Total Fat: 15g; Saturated Fat: 3g; Cholesterol: 18mg; Sodium: 335mg; Total Carbohydrates: 27g; Fiber: 3g; Protein: 12g

Little Fishes, Red Pepper, and Potato Cakes

SERVES 6
Prep time: 15 minutes
Cook time: 20 minutes

1 pound russet, Idaho, or Yukon Gold potatoes (about 3 medium), well scrubbed and cut into ½-inch cubes

1 teaspoon kosher or sea salt

3 (3.75- to 4.25-ounce) tins boneless, skinless sardines in olive oil, drained and oil reserved

1 (12-ounce) jar roasted red peppers, drained, finely chopped, and liquid reserved

½ medium red onion, diced

½ cup chopped fresh parsley, leaves and stems

1 large egg

¼ teaspoon black pepper

¾ cup plain 2% Greek yogurt

1 cup panko or plain bread crumbs

1 tablespoon extra-virgin olive oil

Please don't skip over this recipe once you see sardines in the ingredients. Despite being a lover of all things seafood, Deanna wasn't a fan of those super-sustainable "little fishes" until this dish. Prepped and cooked like crab cakes, the creamy potatoes and sweet bell peppers along with the buttery olive oil all tame the stronger flavor of the sardines. Repurpose the drained sardine oil and the red pepper liquid to whip up a savory yogurt topping—which adds another level of flavor that makes this sardine dish totally crave-worthy.

Put the potatoes in a medium saucepan and pour in cold water to about 1 inch above the potatoes. Add the salt. Cover and bring to a boil over medium-high heat. Reduce the heat to medium and simmer, uncovered, until the potatoes are tender when pierced with a fork, 8 to 10 minutes. Drain and let cool for a few minutes.

While the potatoes cook, gently mash the drained sardines with a fork in a large bowl. Add the red peppers, onion, parsley, egg, and black pepper. Set aside until the potatoes are ready.

Also while the potatoes cook, pour the reserved sardine oil into the jar of red pepper liquid, cover with the lid, and shake to combine. In a small bowl, whisk the yogurt with 1 tablespoon of the oil-pepper liquid mixture and set aside. (For bonus "food saver" points, store the jar of remaining oil-pepper liquid in the refrigerator for up to 5 days. You can use it to flavor soups or pasta dishes, or make more yogurt sauce to use as a dip or sandwich spread.)

Add the cooked potatoes to the sardine mixture and gently mix with your hands or a wooden spoon. Mix in the bread crumbs (the mixture will be very wet). Form into 12 patties about 3 inches in diameter.

Preheat the grill to 400°F, or medium-high heat. Brush two rimmed baking sheets with the olive oil. Arrange the patties on the sheets, then transfer the

continued

sheets to the grill. Using a spatula, gently press down on each patty. Close the lid and grill for 5 minutes, then flip the patties, cover again, and grill for another 5 minutes. (Alternatively, use a large skillet or a griddle pan that spans two stovetop burners and cook the fish cakes in batches over medium-high heat.) Serve the fish cakes with the flavored yogurt sauce. Store any leftover fish cakes in a sealed container in the refrigerator or wrap in parchment, then cover in aluminum foil and freeze.

Healthy Kitchen Hack: Use leftover or stale pita bread to make bread crumbs. Toast the pita and then pulse it in your blender or food processor a few times until fine crumbs form. Mix in 1 teaspoon za'atar for each cup of crumbs to create a Middle Eastern version of flavored bread crumbs. Use these pita bread crumbs for making any kind of seafood or veggie burgers (as here) or sprinkle over hot pasta or grain dishes.

Per Serving (2 fish cakes plus 2 tablespoons yogurt sauce): Calories: 298; Total Fat: 11g; Saturated Fat: 2g; Cholesterol: 99mg; Sodium: 560mg; Total Carbohydrates: 31g; Fiber: 3g; Protein: 19g

"I followed the Healthy Kitchen Hack and made bread crumbs out of whole-wheat pita for these. The richness of the other ingredients masked the sardine flavor!"

—Chris from Chillicothe, OH

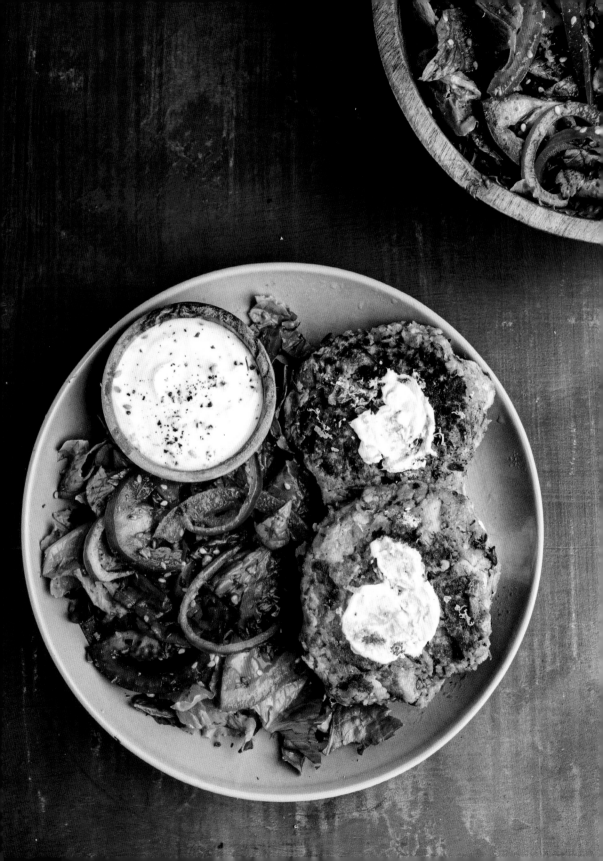

Savory Sardine Tomato Sauce

SERVES 16
Prep time: 5 minutes
Cook time: 30 minutes

2 tablespoons extra-
virgin olive oil

2 (3.75- to 4.25-ounce)
tins boneless, skinless
sardines in olive oil,
undrained

4 garlic cloves,
minced

¼ teaspoon crushed
red pepper (optional)

1 (28-ounce) can
peeled whole tomatoes

1 (28-ounce) can
crushed tomatoes

½ teaspoon dried
oregano

¼ teaspoon kosher or
sea salt

¼ teaspoon black
pepper

¼ teaspoon sugar
(optional)

½ cup fresh basil,
leaves and stems
(optional)

In about half an hour, you can make a robust homemade tomato sauce with canned goods featuring our go-to favorite tinned fish: sardines. Be sure to buy peeled *whole* canned tomatoes (not diced). Whole tomatoes are preferable for sauce-making because they are typically the Roma-style, plum-shaped variety, which have more pulp and less juice. While sardines and tomatoes are a classic Mediterranean combination, we call this a "beginner sardine" sauce to ease those who may be wary into liking these little fishes. Pair with hardy "sauce-loving" pasta shapes like penne, rigatoni, or ziti. (Deanna particularly likes it with gnocchi, like our Homemade Spinach-Ricotta Gnocchi on page 164.) Or use as a base for a thick tomato-based fish stew, adding broth, carrots, potatoes, celery, and/or more canned or frozen seafood.

In a large stockpot over medium heat, heat the olive oil and 1 tablespoon oil from one of the sardine tins. Add the garlic and crushed red pepper (if using) and cook, stirring frequently, for 30 seconds. Reduce the heat to medium-low. Remove the sardines from the tins with a fork and add them to the pot (if you like, save the remaining sardine oil and use it as we suggest in the Hack). Using a wooden spoon, mash and stir frequently for 3 minutes or until the fish resembles the texture of canned tuna (there will be barely any oil left in the pot at this point). Add the whole tomatoes with their juices, crushed tomatoes, oregano, salt, and black pepper. Pour ½ cup water into each empty tomato can, swirl around to get all the remaining juice clinging to the cans, and pour into the pot. Raise the heat to medium and bring to a simmer. Cook, uncovered, for 25 minutes, stirring occasionally and breaking up the whole tomatoes with your wooden spoon. (If the sauce goes above a simmer and starts rapidly bubbling at any point, reduce the heat to medium-low.) Taste the sauce and if you find it too acidic, stir in the sugar.

Gently tear or finely chop the basil leaves and stems if desired, and mix into the sauce. If you're not using the sauce immediately, let it cool for about 15 minutes, then transfer to airtight containers and store in the refrigerator for up to 4 days or in the freezer for up to 6 months.

Healthy Kitchen Hack: Don't throw out the bonus liquid in jarred and canned goods! Throughout this book, we've shared ideas on adding chickpea liquid to hummus, roasted red pepper liquid to soups, olive brine to dressings, and more. Leftover tinned sardine oil is another great flavor enhancer. Store it in a glass jar in the refrigerator for up to 5 days and sauté garlic and onions in it, use as a base for vinaigrette, add along with reserved pasta water to make instant pasta sauce, or mix into any hot grain dish for an extra punch of savory taste.

Per Serving: Calories: 66; Total Fat: 4g; Saturated Fat: 1g; Cholesterol: 16mg; Sodium: 171mg; Total Carbohydrates: 4g; Fiber: 1g; Protein: 4g

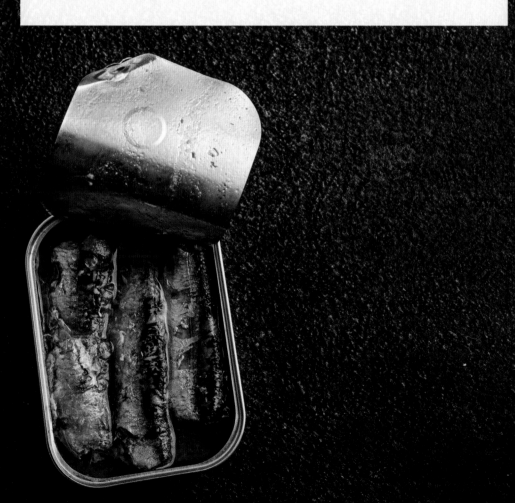

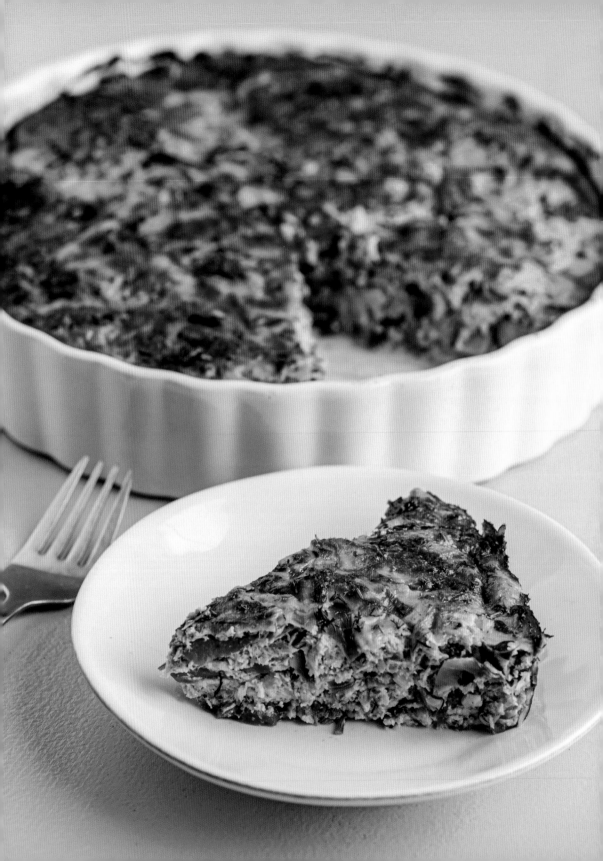

Salmon and Goat Cheese Crustless Qui-ttata

SERVES 6
Prep time: 10 minutes
Cook time: 40 minutes

1 tablespoon extra-virgin olive oil

½ medium red onion, thinly sliced

2 garlic cloves, minced

5 large eggs

½ cup plain 2% Greek yogurt

2 teaspoons balsamic or red wine vinegar

2 teaspoons za'atar

¼ teaspoon kosher or sea salt

¼ teaspoon black pepper

¼ teaspoon crushed red pepper (optional)

4 ounces goat cheese

1 (14.75-ounce) can *or* 3 (5-ounce) cans boneless, skinless salmon, drained

1 (12-ounce) jar roasted red peppers, drained (liquid saved for another use) and sliced

1 cup arugula or spinach

1 cup fresh dill, cilantro, or parsley (or a combination), leaves and stems, finely chopped

Canned salmon perhaps is not as glamorous as a grilled salmon fillet, but its rich and slightly salty taste delivers superb flavor to recipes. Plus, it's a super convenient way to add protein and omega-3s to any meal. Somewhere between a crustless quiche (more dairy than eggs) and a frittata (mainly eggs), this "qui-ttata" is bursting with the colors of leafy greens and herbs plus purple onions and roasted red peppers. But the star ingredients are the combo of salmon and goat cheese (think of the bagel topper: smoked salmon and cream cheese!). Eat this beautiful one-dish meal warm from the oven or cold the next day.

Preheat the oven to 400°F.

Heat the oil in a small skillet over medium heat. Add the onion and cook until starting to brown, about 5 minutes. Add the garlic and cook, stirring frequently, for 1 minute. Remove from the heat.

While the onion cooks, in a large bowl, whisk together the eggs, yogurt, vinegar, za'atar, salt, black pepper, and crushed red pepper (if using). Cut the goat cheese into slabs (to make it easier to mix), add to the bowl, and fold into the ingredients (there will be lumps of goat cheese throughout the egg mixture). Set aside.

In another large bowl, mix together the salmon, roasted red peppers, arugula, herbs, and cooked onion (the heat of the onion will start to wilt the greens). Add the egg mixture and stir until everything is incorporated (again, there will be lumps of goat cheese).

Pour the mixture into a 9-inch pie plate or casserole dish. Bake for 35 minutes or until the center is just set. Remove from the oven and cool on a wire rack for 10 minutes before cutting and serving.

Healthy Kitchen Hack: Like most of our recipes, you can modify this one when you have other ingredients

continued

on hand that you need to use up or just simply want to change up the flavor.

- Instead of salmon: canned tuna, canned sardines, smoked salmon, or smoked trout
- Instead of red onion: white, yellow, or sweet onion; leek; or scallions
- Instead of za'atar: dried oregano and smoked paprika or dried rosemary and dried tarragon
- Instead of arugula/spinach: leftover chopped cooked broccoli, cauliflower, potatoes, squash, or eggplant
- Instead of goat cheese: Made-in-Minutes Homemade Ricotta (page 48), cottage cheese, crumbled feta or Gorgonzola, cubed fresh mozzarella, or any shredded aged cheese (like cheddar or Manchego)
- Instead of roasted red peppers: shredded cabbage, shredded carrots, or any slaw mix

---

Per Serving: Calories: 267; **Total Fat:** 15g; **Saturated Fat:** 5g; **Cholesterol:** 207mg; **Sodium:** 680mg; **Total Carbohydrates:** 8g; **Fiber:** 12g; **Protein:** 26g

"Za'atar was new to me, but I found it easily in my store. The overall dish was colorful and healthy. I had it for lunch the next day and liked it even better served cold!"

—Kate from Houston, TX

Herb-a-licious Baked Clams

SERVES 6
Prep time: 10 minutes
Cook time: 15 minutes

1 tablespoon extra-virgin olive oil

½ medium red onion, diced

2 garlic cloves, minced

6 (6.5-ounce) cans minced or chopped clams, drained and liquid reserved

1 (12-ounce) jar roasted red peppers, drained (liquid saved for another use) and finely chopped

¾ cup panko bread crumbs

½ cup chopped fresh parsley and/or cilantro, leaves and stems

2 tablespoons fresh oregano and/or thyme leaves *or* 2 teaspoons dried oregano and/or thyme

2 tablespoons grated Parmesan or Romano cheese, divided

¼ teaspoon black pepper

⅛–¼ teaspoon crushed red pepper

1 lemon

Next time you drop canned tuna into your shopping cart, expand your seafood horizons and grab some canned clams for your pantry, too. High in protein, iron, selenium, vitamin B12, and vitamin C (to name just a few nutrients), clams are bivalves, which have a minimal environmental impact since they are filter feeders, cleaning waterways while increasing the biodiversity of the ocean. Inspiration for these vibrant baked clams came from Deanna's Nana's Clams Casino, an appetizer she'd serve on the half shell for special occasions and Christmas. But you won't need to go collecting clam shells, since we bake them in ramekins instead. To make a full meal, serve with our Smashed Potatoes with Romesco Sauce on page 91 (boil the potatoes while the clams cook) or serve with baked potatoes and corn on the cob for an indoor clambake.

Preheat the oven to 425°F. Coat six 5- or 6-inch ramekins with cooking spray.

Heat the oil in a large skillet over medium heat. Add the onion and garlic and cook for 1 minute, stirring often. Add ¼ cup of the reserved clam juice (save the remaining for heating up pasta or as a base for Any-Day Bouillabaisse on page 119). Cook for another 4 minutes, stirring occasionally. Remove from the heat and stir in the chopped roasted red peppers.

In a large bowl, mix together the clams, panko, herbs, 1 tablespoon grated cheese, black pepper, and crushed red pepper. Add the onion mixture and mix until all the ingredients are incorporated.

Evenly distribute the clam mixture between the prepared ramekins. Sprinkle the remaining 1 tablespoon grated cheese evenly over all the ramekins.

Place the ramekins on a rimmed baking sheet and bake for 15 minutes. Using a Microplane or citrus zester, grate the zest from the lemon over the ramekins, then cut the lemon into wedges. Serve the baked clams warm with the lemon wedges.

continued

Herb-a-licious Baked Clams *(continued)*

Healthy Kitchen Hack: From switching cooking vessels to seafood swaps, this recipe can be adapted in several sustainable ways. If you have a large enough toaster oven, use it here. Skip cleaning all those ramekins and instead bake the entire clam mixture in a 1-quart baking dish in your oven. Or, use hollowed-out whole tomatoes, bell peppers, or zucchini halves as the cooking "containers." Serve these baked clams over reheated pasta or grains or spoon onto small pieces of toasted bread à la bruschetta. Don't have clams in your pantry? Swap in canned sardines (a yummy way to introduce them into your eating routine!), canned tuna, canned salmon, canned crab, smoked sardines, smoked mackerel, smoked mussels, or any leftover cooked fish.

Per Serving: Calories: 184; Total Fat: 5g; Saturated Fat: 1g; Cholesterol: 124mg; Sodium: 588mg; Total Carbohydrates: 19g; Fiber: 1g; Protein: 18g

"This dish is like taking a quick trip to Cape Cod—and you get all the goodness of stuffed clams without the hassle of the shells."

—Andy from Blue Bell, PA

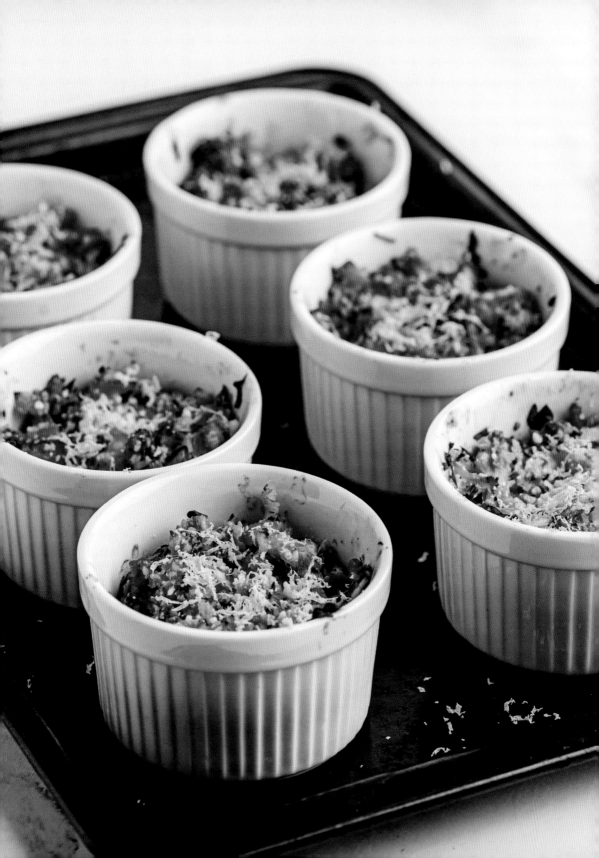

Smoked Seafood Farro "Risotto"

SERVES 6
Prep time: 10 minutes
Cook time: 35 minutes

4 (2.5- to 3.5-ounce) tins smoked trout, smoked oysters, smoked mussels, or any smoked seafood combination, preferably in olive oil (not drained)

1 tablespoon extra-virgin olive oil

1 medium onion (any type), finely chopped

4 garlic cloves, minced

½ teaspoon dried thyme

1½ cups uncooked pearled or 10-minute farro

4 cups Veggie Scraps Broth (page 120), low-sodium vegetable broth, clam juice, or a combination, divided

¼ cup tomato paste

2 teaspoons red wine vinegar or balsamic vinegar

⅓ cup shaved Parmesan or Pecorino Romano cheese (about 1 ounce)

¼ teaspoon black pepper

½ cup finely chopped fresh parsley or cilantro, leaves and stems

Tinned smoked seafood is growing in popularity in the US, and we could not be more excited! From mussels to trout, smoking and canning fish and shellfish shortly after harvesting delivers phenomenal flavor and a long shelf life to a food source that is rarely a local or fresh option. For this riff on risotto, instead of the traditional arborio rice, we use farro, a grain that grows well in poor soil where few other crops thrive. This ancient grain cooks easily and doesn't need constant attention while simmering. Serve warm with crusty bread to mop up the smoky, deep amber–colored sauce and a salad to round out the meal.

Pour 2 tablespoons oil or brine from the smoked seafood into a medium saucepan or stockpot. Add the olive oil and heat over medium heat. Add the onion and cook for 4 minutes or until the onion starts to soften, stirring frequently. Add the garlic and thyme and cook for 30 seconds, stirring frequently. Add the farro and cook for 1 minute, stirring frequently. Add 1 cup broth and cook for 1 minute, stirring occasionally. Add the remaining 3 cups broth and the tomato paste, whisk well, and bring to a boil. Reduce the heat to medium-low and simmer, stirring occasionally, until most of the liquid is absorbed, about 25 minutes. Stir in the vinegar and remove from the heat. Gently mix in the smoked seafood (if using smoked fish, carefully flake into chunks as you stir). Stir in the cheese and pepper. Top with the chopped herbs and serve.

Healthy Kitchen Hack: Instead of reaching for a can of tuna to bulk up a sandwich, salad, pasta, or grain dish, stock your pantry with other yummy tinned smoked seafood options to get more variety and sustainability into your meal routine! Add smoked mussels or oysters to pasta sauce, veggie soups, or leafy green salads. Mix smoked trout, mackerel, or sardines into mayo (or any dressing you mix with tuna) for sandwiches, or add the flaked fish to scrambled eggs or fish cakes, like our Little Fishes, Red Pepper, and Potato Cakes (page 207). Or enjoy one of Serena's favorite snacks, smoked fish on hearty crackers topped with vinegary diced pickles or relish.

Per Serving: Calories: 385; Total Fat: 13g; Saturated Fat: 3g; Cholesterol: 49mg; Sodium: 525mg; Total Carbohydrates: 47g; Fiber: 6g; Protein: 21g

"I was skeptical about adding smoked seafood and using farro for risotto but both gave an entirely new taste dimension, which makes this recipe even better than typical risotto."

—Jim from Havertown, PA

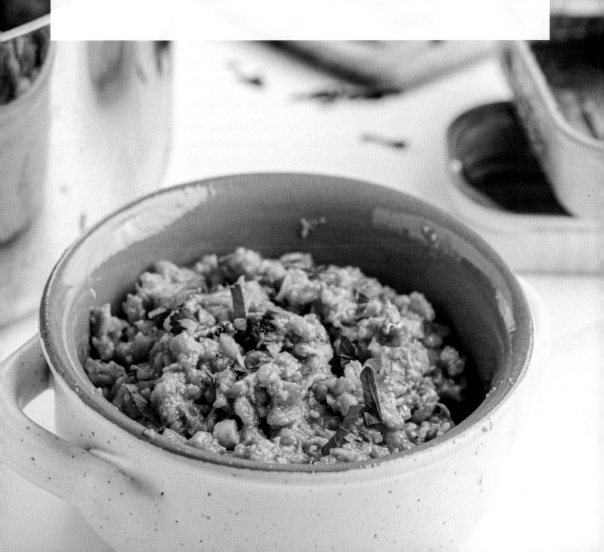

Steamed Mussels with Chorizo and Tomatoes

SERVES 4
Prep time: 10 minutes
Cook time: 20 minutes

2 pounds fresh mussels

2 tablespoons extra-virgin olive oil

1 small onion (any type), chopped

2 celery stalks, finely chopped

2 (4-ounce) links Spanish chorizo sausage or kielbasa, cut into ¼-inch slices

2 garlic cloves, minced

½ teaspoon smoked paprika

½ teaspoon black pepper

1 (15-ounce) can diced tomatoes

¾ cup dry white wine, such as chardonnay or pinot grigio, or Veggie Scraps Broth (page 120)

1 cup chopped fresh parsley or cilantro, leaves and stems

Fresh mussels are not always in our dinner recipe rotation, but for the occasions when we do grab a bag from the fish counter, we are always amazed at how straightforward they are to cook up (not to mention delectable to eat). We hope you'll try these slightly spicy, super aromatic mussels in wine-enriched broth, which is ideal for dunking chunks of crusty bread. They are truly so easy to make: just give them a quick scrub and pop them in a pot. One more point to perhaps convince you to cook them (at least once!) is that they are a highly rated, sustainable seafood choice and actually help improve the ocean environment.

In a large colander in the sink, run cold water over the mussels (but don't let the mussels sit in standing water or ice). Use a stiff brush to scrub off any barnacles or sand (see Note). All the shells should be closed tight (if a few are open, tap them, they should close, indicating they're alive); discard any shells that stay open or are cracked. Leave the mussels in the colander until you're ready to use them.

Heat the oil in a large Dutch oven or stockpot over medium heat. Add the onion and celery and cook, stirring occasionally, until they start to soften, about 5 minutes. Add the chorizo, garlic, smoked paprika, and pepper; cook, stirring occasionally, for 6 to 8 minutes until the chorizo begins to brown in spots. Add the tomatoes with their juices, wine, and mussels, cover, and steam for 3 to 5 minutes, until the mussels open their shells. Gently shake the pot once or twice while they cook. With a slotted spoon, discard any mussels that don't open. Top with the parsley and serve from the pot using a soup ladle to get broth into each bowl. Put out an empty bowl for discarded shells. For any leftover mussels, remove the meat from the shells, cover with broth, and store in an airtight container in the refrigerator for up to 24 hours or in the freezer for up to 4 months.

Note: Nearly all the mussels found at seafood counters come debearded. However, if you happen to see hair-like fibers attached to the shell, just pull off the "beard."

Healthy Kitchen Hack: Instead of tossing those mussel shells, you can actually compost them (they will break down). If you live by the sea, some marine rehabilitation groups have shell recycling programs and collect them to help rebuild reefs or for repopulating. But before they leave your kitchen, you can freeze and use them in our Fish Stock recipe (page 203). Or if you're feeling creative, you can scrub them with soap and water, dry them, and use them for crafts. (Deanna has painted mussel, clam, and oyster shells over the years and has even glued them to frames and mirrors!)

Per Serving: Calories: 257; Total Fat: 18g; Saturated Fat: 5g; Cholesterol: 30mg; Sodium: 427mg; Total Carbohydrates: 9g; Fiber: 3g; Protein: 9g

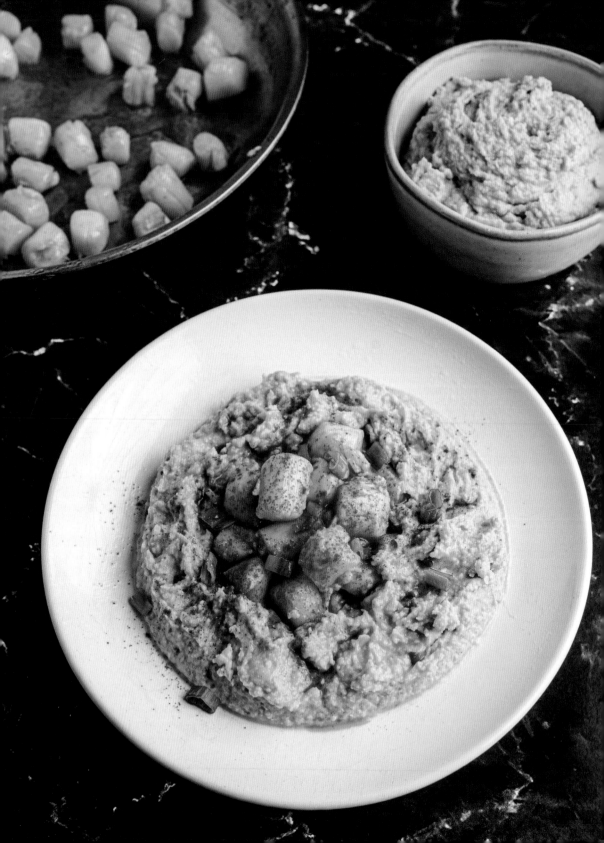

Seared Bay Scallops with Baby Lima Bean Puree

SERVES 4

Prep time: 10 minutes
Cook time: 10 minutes

1 (1-pound) bag frozen baby lima beans

1 (1-pound) bag frozen bay scallops, thawed

½ teaspoon smoked paprika, divided, plus more for garnish if desired

½ teaspoon kosher or sea salt, divided

½ teaspoon black pepper, divided

4 tablespoons extra-virgin olive oil, divided

4 scallions (green onions), green and white parts, thinly sliced
Save the stems!
See page 70

1 lemon

The great news about succulent, sweet bay scallops is they are a sustainable, aquaculture farmed option. But unless you live by the coast, it's next to impossible to get them fresh. Solution: frozen bay scallops. These tiny gems can be whipped up into a simple yet gourmet meal in minutes, and bonus, they're typically less than half the price of larger sea scallops. This scallop recipe was adapted from an old Teaspoon of Spice blog post that Deanna threw together when she got fresh fava beans in her farm share. While brainstorming about an easy and accessible swap, Serena suggested baby lima beans. Deanna balked at first (she's never been a fan) but is glad she put her lima bean prejudices aside because these little guys worked like a charm in a puree that reminds us of a fresher, lighter hummus in taste and texture.

Cook the baby lima beans on the stove in water according to the package directions. Drain, saving the cooking water in a bowl (should be around ¼ cup), and return the beans to the pot.

While the beans cook, pat dry the thawed scallops with a dish towel. Sprinkle with ¼ teaspoon each smoked paprika, salt, and pepper.

Heat 2 tablespoons oil in a large skillet over medium heat. Add half of the scallops and cook, gently stirring almost constantly, until milky white and firm, 2½ to 4 minutes (depending on their size and package instructions). Using tongs or a slotted spoon, transfer the cooked scallops to a small bowl. Repeat with the remaining scallops.

Return the skillet to the stove and add the reserved bean cooking water and about three-quarters of the sliced scallions. Using a Microplane or citrus zester, grate the zest from the lemon into the skillet; cut the lemon in half and squeeze in the juice. Cook over medium heat, scraping up any browned bits to make a sauce, about 2 minutes. Remove from the heat.

continued

To make the puree, pour the drained beans into a high-powered blender or food processor. Add the lemon skillet sauce, remaining 2 tablespoons oil, and remaining ¼ teaspoon each smoked paprika, salt, and pepper. Pour in ⅓ cup water and start to puree. Add more water, 1 tablespoon at a time, until the puree reaches a hummus-like consistency.

To serve, divide the lima bean puree among four plates. Spoon the scallops over the puree, then drizzle with any scallop juice left in the bowl. Sprinkle each plate with remaining sliced scallion and dust with extra smoked paprika if desired.

Healthy Kitchen Hack: While Deanna would *now* encourage you to stock baby lima beans in your freezer (if you don't already), you can also swap in other frozen or canned legumes here. Try frozen peas, frozen fava beans, canned chickpeas, or canned great northern beans. Or mix up the spice flavors by subbing in za'atar, fennel seeds, or everything bagel seasoning for the smoked paprika.

Per Serving: Calories: 307; Total Fat: 15g; Saturated Fat: 2g; Cholesterol: 4mg; Sodium: 487mg; Total Carbohydrates: 22g; Fiber: 5g; Protein: 24g

Spicy Fish Shawarma Bowls

SERVES 2
Prep time: 10 minutes
Cook time: 5 minutes

Shawarma is a popular Middle Eastern sandwich of slow-cooked seasoned meat (like beef, goat, chicken, or lamb) that's shaved and piled onto pita or flatbread. While it may sound like a Greek gyro, the difference is in the distinct spices and the array of colorful pickled toppers to choose from. Nowadays, you'll see all types of variations beyond the typical sandwich; in fact, when Deanna visited Israel, she enjoyed a fish shawarma entrée that was plated on a bed of herbs and a swirl of spicy sauce. Here we've recreated the aromatic and enticing spice blend that makes this a street food classic, then sprinkled it over white fish, and served it up in a deconstructed bowl style along with an assembly of traditional condiments. Feel free to swap in your favorite accompaniments, then check out the other ways to enjoy your new shawarma spice mix in this recipe's Healthy Kitchen Hack.

1 teaspoon ground cinnamon

1 teaspoon ground coriander

1 teaspoon ground cumin

1 teaspoon ground turmeric

¾ teaspoon paprika

½ teaspoon garlic powder

⅛ teaspoon cayenne pepper or crushed red pepper

⅛ teaspoon black pepper

6 ounces cooked *or* 8 ounces uncooked white fish fillets (from the More Sustainable Seafood Choices list on page 19) *or* 6 ounces canned seafood

¼ teaspoon kosher or sea salt (optional)

2 teaspoons extra-virgin olive oil (optional)

1 cup Antipasto Pickles (page 52) or store-bought pickles

1 cup Toasted Cauliflower Tabbouleh (page 96), cooked bulgur, or cooked couscous

½ cup coarsely chopped cucumber

1 large whole-wheat pita bread, cut into wedges

¼ cup plus 2 tablespoons Lemon Hummus (page 231) or tahini

To make the shawarma spice mix, in a small mixing bowl, whisk together the cinnamon, coriander, cumin, turmeric, paprika, garlic powder, cayenne pepper, and black pepper.

If using cooked fish, flake the fish in a microwave-safe bowl and sprinkle with 1 teaspoon shawarma spice mix. Reheat in the microwave for 20 seconds. Sprinkle with the salt.

If using uncooked fish, pour the olive oil into a glass pie dish or large microwave-safe bowl. Pat the fillets dry and season with the salt. Flip the fillets in the oil a few times until coated. Cover the dish with a microwave-safe plate and microwave on high for 2½ minutes. Carefully remove the hot dish with oven mitts and let some

continued

of the steam escape before removing the plate. Check the fillet with a fork to see if the fish is just starting to separate into flakes. If any part doesn't look cooked, cover again and microwave in 20-second increments until done. Once the fish is cooked, sprinkle with 1 teaspoon shawarma spice mix and gently flake to fully season it throughout.

If using canned fish, sprinkle with 1 teaspoon shawarma spice mix, flake, and mix; skip the heating and salting steps.

To assemble the shawarma bowls, arrange the seasoned fish, pickles, tabbouleh, cucumber, and pita pieces in sections in a soup or dinner bowl. Dollop the hummus on top in the middle of the bowl.

Healthy Kitchen Hack: Since this shawarma spice mix recipe yields close to 2 tablespoons total, you'll have plenty left over to make more shawarma bowls. Or, store it in a recycled spice jar and also use it to flavor:

- Vegetables before roasting

- Kebabs of any kind

- Tofu before baking or frying

- Chili and stews (in place of chili powder)

- Popcorn (add some salt)

- Plain yogurt for a savory sauce or dip

- Canned beans for soups, hummus, pasta, and other grain dishes

---

Per Serving: Calories: 359; Total Fat: 13g; Saturated Fat: 1g; Cholesterol: 63mg; Sodium: 789mg; Total Carbohydrates: 36g; Fiber: 7g; Protein: 25g

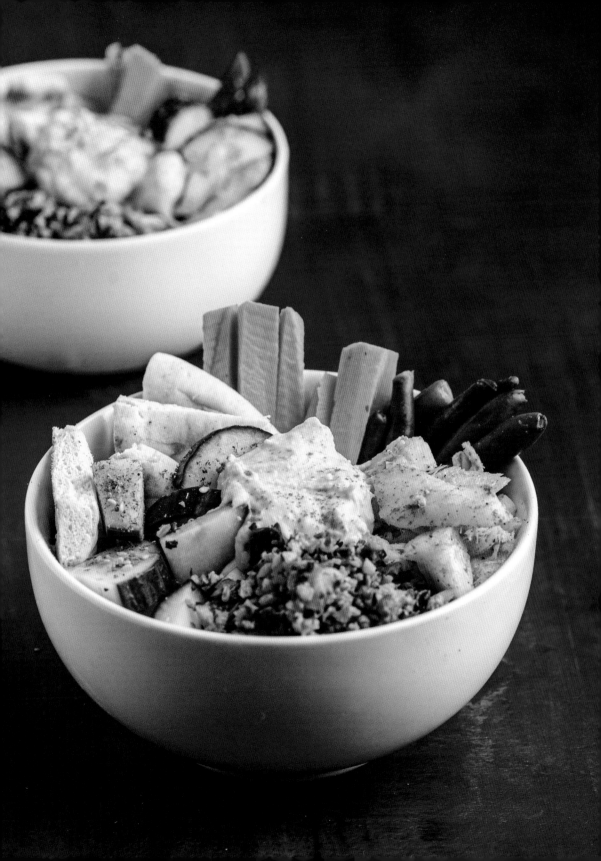

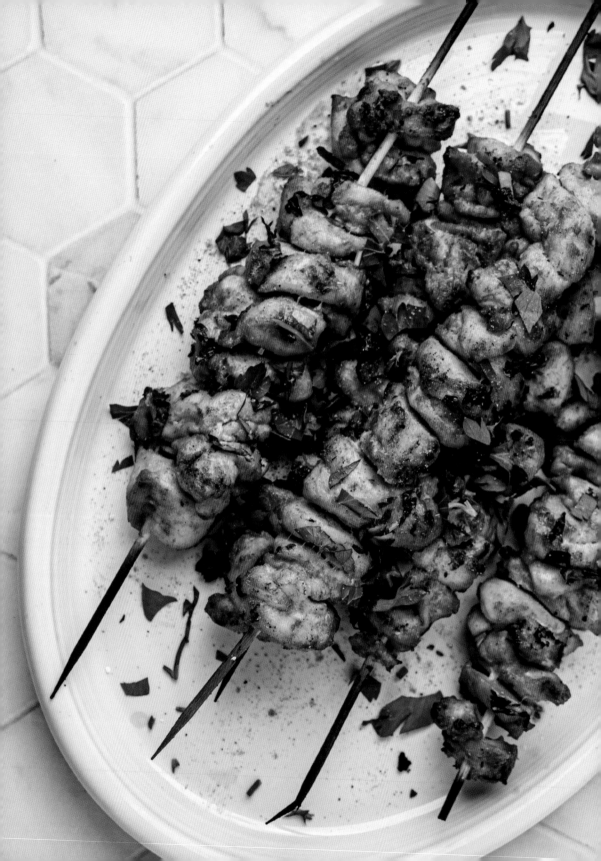

Meats and Poultry

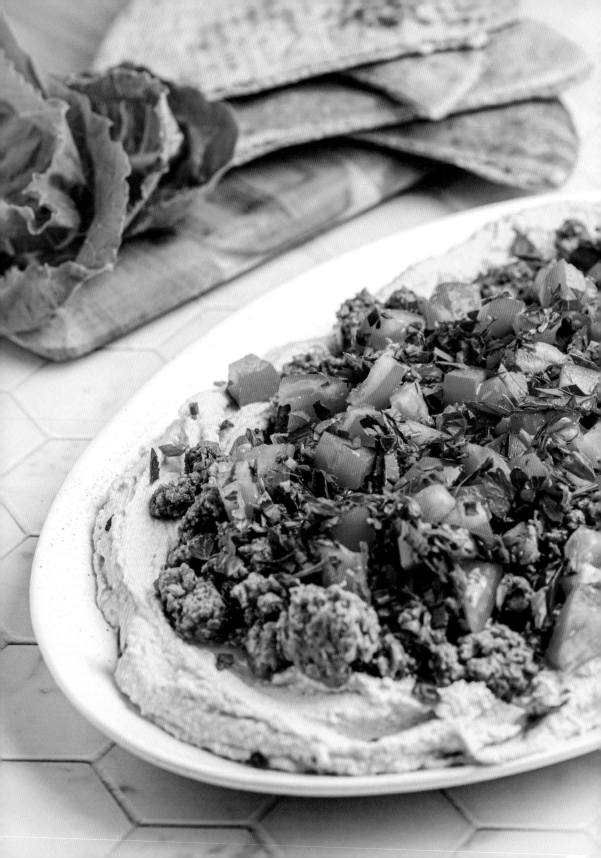

Spiced Ground Beef over Lemon Hummus

SERVES 8

Prep time: 15 minutes
Cook time: 15 minutes

8 ounces white button mushrooms

½ medium onion (any type), quartered

5 tablespoons extra-virgin olive oil, divided

2 garlic cloves, minced

1 teaspoon za'atar

½ teaspoon kosher or sea salt, divided

¼ teaspoon black pepper

¼ teaspoon smoked paprika

1 pound ground beef (80 to 90% lean)

2 lemons

2 (15-ounce) cans chickpeas, drained and liquid reserved

¼ cup tahini or peanut butter

1 cup chopped tomatoes or drained canned diced tomatoes

¾–1 cup chopped cilantro or parsley, leaves and stems

Pita bread and/or romaine lettuce leaves, for dipping and wrapping (optional)

Here's a new way to look at ground beef! First, we use our budget-friendly trick of extending it and making the dish more plant-forward by mincing and mixing in cooked mushrooms, which have a meaty umami flavor. The warm beef and mushroom mixture is seasoned with Mediterranean spices and served in the classic Middle Eastern way: brought to the table over a bed of creamy homemade hummus (made by you in less than 10 minutes!). It's all topped off with tomatoes and herbs, then served with pita bread for scooping. Or, if you need to keep the meal gluten-free, serve with leafy greens to stuff, roll, and wrap.

In a food processor or blender, pulse half of the mushrooms and half of the onion quarters about 10 times or until the mushrooms and onion are minced, resembling the same texture as ground beef. Remove and repeat with the remaining mushrooms and onion quarters.

Heat 1 tablespoon oil in a large skillet over medium heat. Add all the minced mushrooms and onion and cook, stirring occasionally, until the mushrooms start to wilt, about 5 minutes. Add the garlic, za'atar, ¼ teaspoon salt, pepper, and smoked paprika and cook, stirring frequently, for 1 minute. Add the ground beef and cook, breaking up the chunks with a wooden spoon and stirring occasionally, until the beef is cooked through and is no longer pink, about 8 minutes. Remove from the heat.

While the beef cooks, make the hummus. Using a Microplane or citrus zester, grate the zest from the lemons over your rinsed-out food processor or blender, then cut the lemons in half and squeeze in the juice. Add the chickpeas, 6 tablespoons reserved chickpea liquid, remaining ¼ cup oil, tahini, and remaining ¼ teaspoon salt. Process until smooth, adding another tablespoon or two of the reserved chickpea liquid to adjust the consistency to your preference.

continued

To serve, spread the lemon hummus on a large serving platter. Top with the warm ground beef-mushroom mixture and then the tomatoes. Sprinkle the herbs over the top and serve with pita and/or romaine leaves if desired.

Note: Peanut butter may be substituted for tahini, but the recipe will no longer be nut-free.

Healthy Kitchen Hack: Adapt the recipe to what you have on hand! Add extra mushrooms to the blender or use ground turkey instead of ground beef. Experiment with different spices in the beef-mushroom mixture, like ground coriander, cumin, allspice, turmeric, or cayenne pepper. Or use up any extra fresh cilantro, parsley, basil, or mint lurking in your fridge by adding them to the blender to make a "green" hummus.

Per Serving (without pita or lettuce): Calories: 336; Total Fat: 21g; Saturated Fat: 4g; Cholesterol: 38mg; Sodium: 432mg; Total Carbohydrates: 21g; Fiber: 6g; Protein: 19g

"My whole family loved this. My daughter said it would also make a great appetizer. And the lemon hummus is amazing—I'd make that all by itself!"

—Alli from Plymouth, MI

Stuffed Greek Lamb Burgers

SERVES 4
Prep time: 20 minutes
Cook time: 10 minutes

1 pound ground lamb

½ teaspoon garlic powder

½ teaspoon kosher or sea salt, divided

¼ teaspoon black pepper

1 medium red onion

¼ cup crumbled feta cheese

½ cup plain 2% Greek yogurt

2 teaspoons extra-virgin olive oil

1 cucumber

¼ cup chopped fresh mint, leaves and stems

4 lettuce leaves

4 tomato slices

4 whole-wheat burger buns or pita breads

"The feta filling certainly sets these burgers apart from all the rest. Delicious!"

—Lindsey from Havertown, PA

Prepare to love lamb! Lamb is adored all over the Mediterranean, and American lamb is pasture-raised on land that's otherwise pretty unsuitable for crops. Lamb ranchers turn "scrub" land into protein for our plates that's rich in yummy umami and heart-healthy monounsaturated fats. Filled with salty feta and tangy onion, these bold burgers are topped with a cool minty yogurt spread that makes for one giant sandwich. Enjoy them stacked up high in buns, stuffed into pita bread, or even on their own. Any way you serve them, we think you'll find your new favorite burger.

Line a large rimmed baking sheet with aluminum foil. Arrange the top oven rack about 4 inches from the broiler. Preheat the broiler to high.

In a large bowl, gently mix together the lamb, garlic powder, ¼ teaspoon salt, and pepper with your hands. Measure out ¼ cup of the lamb mixture and set aside. Divide the remaining lamb mixture into four equal portions and shape each portion into a burger about ¾ inch thick. Gently press your fingers into the center of each burger to make a ¼-inch-deep indentation about 1 inch in diameter. Transfer the burgers to a plate and set aside.

Slice four thin slices from the onion and set them aside for burger assembly. From the remaining onion, dice up 3 tablespoons (save the remaining onion for another use).

In a small bowl, using a fork, mash and mix together the feta and diced onion to make the burger filling. Divide the filling among the burgers and press gently into the center indentations. Flatten 1 tablespoon of the reserved meat over the burger filling on one of the filled patties, pinching the edges to seal; repeat with the remaining 3 tablespoons meat and the remaining burgers. Transfer to the prepared baking sheet.

Broil the burgers for 4 minutes, flip them, and continue broiling until the internal temperature of the meat (not the filling) is 160°F on a meat thermometer, an

continued

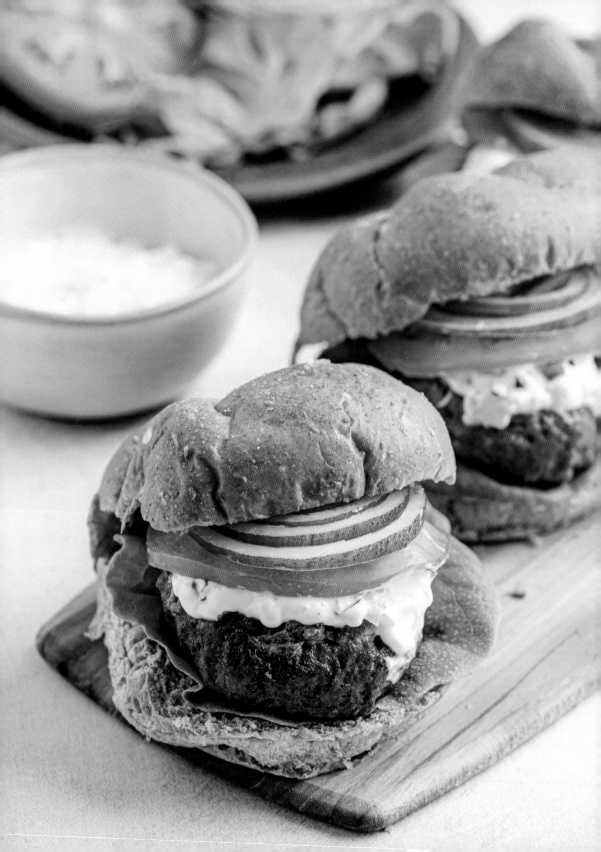

additional 3 to 4 minutes. Your broiler may flare up or start to smoke because of the close proximity to this rich meat; if this happens, simply open the oven door a crack to lower the oven temperature for 5 to 10 seconds.

While the burgers cook, make the topping. In a medium bowl, whisk together the yogurt, oil, and remaining ¼ teaspoon salt. Cut the cucumber in half. Dice one half and add it to the yogurt mixture. Either save the other half of the cucumber for another use or slice it and set aside for serving. Add the mint to the yogurt mixture and stir everything to combine.

To serve, top each burger with the yogurt mixture, a lettuce leaf, a tomato slice, and an onion slice, and serve on buns with the sliced cucumber on the side if desired.

Healthy Kitchen Hack: We affectionately refer to this yogurt, olive oil, and salt topping as "Mediterranean mayo" as we use the tangy topping on just about everything. It can be a sandwich spread, a salad dressing when made pourable with a bit more olive oil, a marinade for pork or chicken, and even a tartar sauce substitute for fish. Also try dressing up the mayo with herbs and spices, like mixing in ground cumin to top on baked sweet potatoes, fresh basil to smear on any sandwich, or za'atar for an instant dip.

Per Serving (burger alone): Calories: 357; Total Fat: 27g; Saturated Fat: 12g; Cholesterol: 91mg; Sodium: 403mg; Total Carbohydrates: 4g; Fiber: 1g; Protein: 24g

Cumin-Marinated Steak with Charred Peppers and Onions

SERVES 4
Prep time: 30 minutes
Cook time: 20 minutes

2 tablespoons extra-virgin olive oil, divided

2 tablespoons red wine vinegar

1 teaspoon Worcestershire sauce or less-sodium soy sauce

½ teaspoon ground cumin

½ teaspoon smoked paprika

½ teaspoon garlic powder

½ teaspoon kosher or sea salt

½ teaspoon black pepper

1 pound charcoal or flat iron steak

2 large bell peppers (any color), seeded and cut into 8 wedges each

1 large onion, cut into 8 wedges

Meat can occasionally fit into a sustainable Mediterranean Diet (see pages 18–21), and one way to do it is to purchase the less "in-demand" cuts of beef. For instance, the lesser-known charcoal steak (also known, ironically, as a chicken steak) is the most tender cut after the pricier tenderloin, plus it's buttery and flavorful because it's cut from the shoulder blade. Your best chance to find it is in a store where a butcher breaks down a whole animal (see our Hack) or, as a backup, buy a similar cut of flat iron steak. We marinate it with Mediterranean spices for 30 minutes to kick up the flavor, then serve it up with a classic combo of blistered peppers and onions, which take only a few minutes under the broiler, instead of double the cooking time when sautéed on the stovetop.

In a large bowl, whisk together 1 tablespoon oil, the vinegar, Worcestershire sauce, cumin, smoked paprika, garlic powder, salt, and black pepper. Add the meat and turn to coat with the marinade; let sit at room temperature for 30 minutes while you prepare the vegetables.

Arrange the top oven rack about 4 inches from the broiler. Preheat the broiler to high. Coat a large rimmed baking sheet with cooking spray.

Put the bell peppers and onion on the prepared baking sheet and drizzle with the remaining 1 tablespoon oil; toss with your hands to coat. Broil for 5 minutes, then remove the sheet from the oven and flip the vegetables, moving those that are beginning to brown to the edges so they cook evenly. Broil for an additional 5 minutes, watching carefully until the vegetables turn dark brown. Remove the sheet from the oven and remove any bell peppers and onions that appear cooked through; leave the rest on the sheet. Clear a section in the center for the meat and carefully transfer the steak to the hot baking sheet. Broil for 5 minutes, then flip the steak and remove or rearrange any remaining vegetables if they need to cook longer so they will evenly brown. Broil for 3 to 5 more minutes or until the internal temperature of the steak reaches the butcher-recommended medium-rare doneness of 120°F to 130°F on a meat thermometer (or, if you prefer, 135°F to 140°F for medium).

To serve, cut the steak across the grain into thin strips and remove the line of gristle (see Hack). Toss the vegetables in the flavorful meat juices on the baking sheet and serve with the steak.

Healthy Kitchen Hack: If you're a meat eater, chatting with your local butcher is an informative way to discover underappreciated cuts that are tasty and budget-friendly—and might go to waste if they didn't end up in your shopping cart. Serena's butcher has introduced her to less-popular yet still tasty cuts like the oyster, Denver, sirloin flap, coulotte, and merlot. Butchers can also share tips like the fact that charcoal steak has a line of gristle, but it's easy to cut away after cooking.

Per Serving: **Calories: 307; Total Fat: 18g; Saturated Fat: 4g; Cholesterol: 68mg; Sodium: 320mg; Total Carbohydrates: 9g; Fiber: 3g; Protein: 28g**

Spicy Red Lentil and Chorizo Stew

SERVES 4
Prep time: 10 minutes
Cook time: 20 minutes

1 cup dried red lentils, rinsed

3 (4-ounce) Yukon Gold or other potatoes, well scrubbed and cut into ¼-inch cubes

3 tablespoons extra-virgin olive oil, divided

1 onion (any type), chopped

1 yellow or green bell pepper, seeded and chopped

2 (4-ounce) links Spanish chorizo sausage or kielbasa, cut into ¼-inch slices

3 garlic cloves, minced

1½ teaspoons smoked paprika

½ teaspoon black pepper

1 (15-ounce) can low-sodium diced tomatoes

3 tablespoons red wine vinegar

1 cup chopped fresh parsley, leaves and stems

Even if you are spicy-heat timid, don't shy away from trying this Spanish-style stew! It's got the best type of heat: a warming, slightly smoky zestiness that makes you want to keep spooning up more. In the words of Serena's "super-taster" daughter (who isn't a fan of very spicy food), "Mom, I didn't know this was spicy until I finished my whole bowl and it made me feel all warm." That's the magic of smoked paprika, the classic Spanish spice made by smoking peppers over oak wood and then grinding them down. When combined with a little bit of chorizo and two inexpensive and always-in-season ingredients—potatoes and quick-cooking red lentils—this recipe may become one of your new year-round favorite meals.

In a large saucepan or Dutch oven, combine the lentils, potatoes, and 3½ cups water. Bring to a simmer over medium-high heat, then reduce to medium. Simmer, stirring occasionally, until the lentils and potatoes are tender but still hold their shape, about 15 minutes.

While the lentils cook, heat 2 tablespoons oil in a large skillet over medium heat. Add the onion and bell pepper; cook, stirring occasionally, until they start to soften, about 5 minutes. Add the sausage, garlic, smoked paprika, and black pepper and cook, stirring occasionally, until the sausage begins to brown in spots, 6 to 8 minutes. Add the tomatoes with their juices and vinegar and bring to a boil, scraping up any browned bits. Boil for 1 minute. Pour the tomato-sausage mixture into the cooked lentils. Stir in the parsley, drizzle with the remaining 1 tablespoon oil, and serve right out of the pot.

Healthy Kitchen Hack: We know that not everyone loves leftovers (Deanna's husband is in that camp), so here are a few tricks to make extra servings of this stew (or similar recipes) loveable:

- Serve over toast: Reheat, then pour over a piece of crusty bread—eat with a fork and knife!

- Add nuts and/or cheese: Reheat, then mix in creamy goat cheese or feta and/or sprinkle with a few pistachios or walnuts.
- Stir into eggs: When you have one serving of stew, stretch it out by adding it to warm scrambled eggs to feed the whole family.

Per Serving: Calories: 339; Total Fat: 15g; Saturated Fat: 4g; Cholesterol: 20mg; Sodium: 366mg; Total Carbohydrates: 38g; Fiber: 7g; Protein: 15g

"I served it to my friend, who liked the lentils, chorizo, and spice so much that she told her friend about it. Then, *her* friend actually asked for the recipe!"

—Candace from Alhambra, IL

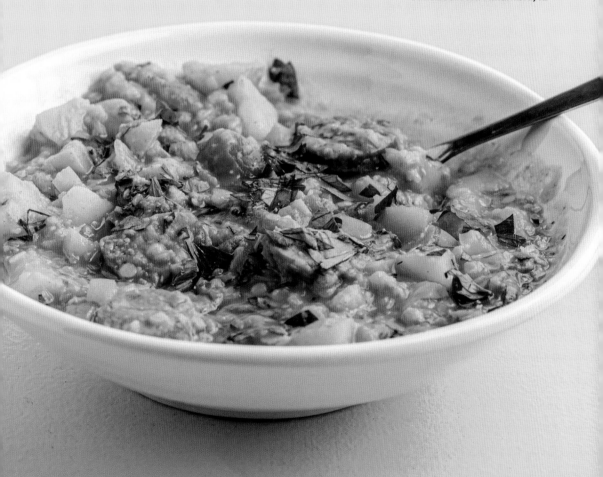

Parsley, Pistachio, and Bulgur Beef Koftas

SERVES 6
Prep time: 10 minutes
Cook time: 15 minutes

½ cup uncooked bulgur

1 cup chopped fresh parsley and/or mint, leaves and stems, plus more for serving if desired

½ cup shelled unsalted pistachios

2 garlic cloves, peeled

½ teaspoon ground cinnamon

½ teaspoon ground coriander

½ teaspoon ground cumin

¼ teaspoon smoked paprika

¼ teaspoon kosher or sea salt

¼ teaspoon black pepper

⅛ teaspoon cayenne pepper

1 pound ground beef (80 to 90% lean)

1 tablespoon extra-virgin olive oil

Across the Mediterranean, there are endless versions of koftas—meatballs that vary in shape, seasonings, cooking methods, and serving styles. Here we extend the ground beef with easy-to-cook bulgur and chopped pistachios, then pack them with parsley, mint, and spices, shape them, and bake them. You may not go back to your regular meatball recipe after tasting these! Wrap the koftas with pita or lettuce leaves and top with our Pumpkin Hummus (page 63) or with plain yogurt.

Preheat the oven to 400°F.

In a small saucepan, bring ½ cup water to a boil over medium-high heat. Add the bulgur and stir once. Cover, reduce the heat to medium-low, and simmer for 10 to 12 minutes or until the liquid is absorbed. Uncover and let cool for about 5 minutes.

While the bulgur cooks, in a food processor, process the herbs, pistachios, garlic, cinnamon, coriander, cumin, smoked paprika, salt, black pepper, and cayenne pepper until a paste forms. Spoon the mixture into a large mixing bowl. Add the cooked bulgur and ground beef. Using your hands, gently mix all the ingredients together (be careful not to overmix).

Divide the mixture into 12 portions and shape into logs about 4 inches long. Transfer to a large rimmed baking sheet and brush with the oil. Bake for 12 to 14 minutes or until the koftas just start to get golden brown and the internal temperature measures 160°F using a meat thermometer.

Serve the koftas warm, sprinkled with extra fresh herbs if desired.

Healthy Kitchen Hack: Instead of bulgur, add other "extenders" to ground meat or poultry. Try cooked couscous, cooked lentils, mashed canned cannellini beans, or cooked minced mushrooms.

Per Serving: Calories: 256; Total Fat: 15g; Saturated Fat: 4g; Cholesterol: 49mg; Sodium: 137mg; Total Carbohydrates: 13g; Fiber: 3g; Protein: 19g

Oregano, Fennel, and Garlic Slow Cooker Pulled Pork

SERVES 10
Prep time: 10 minutes
Cook time: 5 or 10 hours

1 tablespoon dried oregano

2 teaspoons garlic powder

1 teaspoon fennel seeds

1 teaspoon kosher or sea salt

½ teaspoon black pepper

1 (4- to 5-pound) boneless blade pork roast

Boneless blade pork roast—also called pork butt or Boston butt—is perfect for low-and-slow heat. It's one of the most inexpensive and overlooked cuts of pork, so if you've never cooked one, we wouldn't be surprised. Cook it with this simple rub of just five spices, including a Mediterranean darling: sweet anise-flavored fennel seeds. When brainstorming this recipe, we had plans to add a sauce and lots of toppings. But Serena's family loved it straight from the cooker, no extras required.

In a small bowl, combine the oregano, garlic powder, fennel, salt, and pepper. Rub the seasonings all over the pork roast.

Coat the inside of a 5- to 7-quart slow cooker with cooking spray. Place the pork inside with the fat layer side down (if there is a fat layer). Cover and cook on high for 5 hours or on low for 8 to 10 hours, until the pork is very tender.

Using tongs, transfer the pork onto a cutting board. Once cool enough to handle, use two forks (or your fingers) to shred the pork.

While the pork cools, strain the fat from the pork juices using the method in this recipe's Hack. Serve the shredded pork and the pork juices at room temperature (or warmed in the slow cooker on high for 10 minutes).

Healthy Kitchen Hack: Here's a quick way to remove the fat from the pan juices that remain after cooking. Carefully pour the juices from the cooking vessel into a large liquid measuring cup or a pitcher (larger than 2 cups). Cool the juices by placing the pitcher in a bowl large enough to surround it with ice and some water. Cool for at least 10 minutes. Then, using a large spoon, spoon off most of the fat (and reserve in a jar in the refrigerator for flavoring cooked vegetables).

Per Serving: Calories: 303; Total Fat: 13g; Saturated Fat: 5g; Cholesterol: 133mg; Sodium: 251mg; Total Carbohydrates: 1g; Fiber: 0g; Protein: 41g

Chicken Spanako-Pita Bake

SERVES 6
Prep time: 10 minutes
Cook time: 30 minutes

1 (1-pound) package frozen spinach, thawed overnight or barely defrosted in the microwave

1 lemon

2 (12.5-ounce) cans chicken, drained, rinsed, and flaked

1 cup 2% cottage cheese

2 large eggs

2 scallions (green onions), green and white parts, thinly sliced
Save the stems!
See page 70

3 teaspoons dried oregano or dill, divided

¾ teaspoon garlic powder, divided

½ teaspoon black pepper

⅓ cup crumbled feta cheese

1 large whole-wheat pita bread or any leftover flatbread

1 teaspoon extra-virgin olive oil

During her college years, Serena was lucky enough to wait tables at a Greek restaurant run by a talented immigrant family who cooked their traditional recipes from scratch. Whenever one of the cooks pulled a hot tray of flaky, phyllo dough–covered spanakopita (which is Greek for "spinach pie") from the oven, Serena could hardly wait to enjoy a slice. Here, you'll find all the flavors of the traditional filling with spinach, eggs, feta cheese, garlic, and oregano, amped up with tender flaked chicken. But we've simplified the spanakopita making process: instead of layering our filling with temperamental phyllo dough, we top it with crisped-up triangles of pita bread. If you don't usually buy canned chicken, this is the recipe that will convince you it's a terrific shelf-stable ingredient worth keeping on hand (learn more in this recipe's Healthy Kitchen Hack).

Preheat the oven to 375°F. Coat a 9-inch square baking dish or 2-quart casserole dish with cooking spray.

Put the spinach in a colander set over a large bowl and use a silicone scraper to press down on the spinach to remove as much liquid as possible. (Save it for stirring into soups, stews, or smoothies.)

Using a Microplane or citrus zester, grate the zest from the lemon over another large bowl; cut the lemon in half and squeeze in the juice. Add the spinach, chicken, cottage cheese, eggs, scallions, 2½ teaspoons oregano, ½ teaspoon garlic powder, and pepper and mix well. Transfer the mixture to the prepared baking dish. Sprinkle with the feta cheese.

Using kitchen shears or a knife, slit the pita all the way around the edges, open and pull apart so you have two rounds. Brush the outside of the two pita rounds with the oil and sprinkle evenly with the remaining ½ teaspoon oregano and remaining ¼ teaspoon garlic powder. Cut each round into 8 wedges. Arrange the wedges, coated-side up, on top of the spinach mixture so that most of the spanakopita is covered.

Bake for 25 to 30 minutes or until the juices are bubbling and the pita pieces are crisp and lightly browned.

Healthy Kitchen Hack: Like other canned foods, canned chicken is a favorite pantry staple to help prevent food waste. We hate to admit it, but there have certainly been times when our raw chicken was refrigerated longer than recommended for freshness and had to be tossed. Canned chicken is your insurance against this. Drain and rinse it in a colander to remove up to 40 percent of the sodium and then enjoy it in place of canned tuna for sandwiches, wraps, salads, soups, or casseroles, or add to omelets, frittatas, quiches, or tacos.

Per Serving: Calories: 232; Total Fat: 8g; Saturated Fat: 3g; Cholesterol: 134mg; Sodium: 633mg; Total Carbohydrates: 13g; Fiber: 3g; Protein: 29g

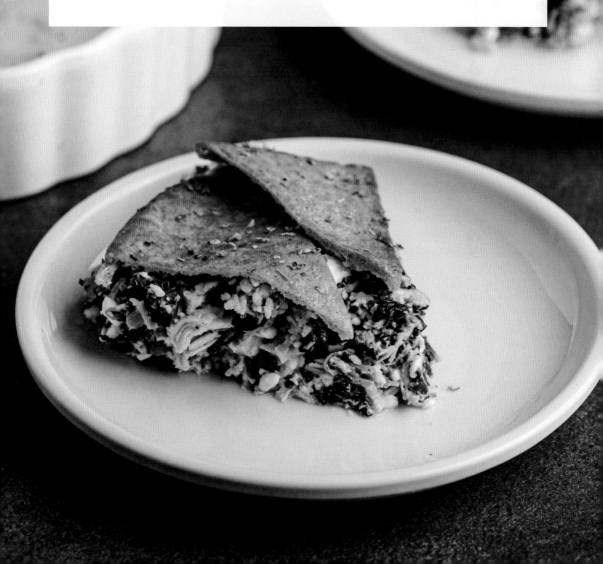

Lemon Chicken Tenders with Capers

SERVES 6
Prep time: 10 minutes
Cook time: 15 minutes

2 lemons

¼ cup yellow cornmeal

2 tablespoons whole-wheat flour, white whole-wheat flour, or all-purpose flour

½ teaspoon kosher or sea salt

½ teaspoon black pepper, divided

3 (8-ounce) boneless, skinless chicken breasts, cut lengthwise into ½-inch-thick strips

3 tablespoons extra-virgin olive oil, divided

¼ cup dry white wine *or* 2 tablespoons white wine vinegar plus 2 tablespoons water

2 tablespoons capers, drained

½ cup chopped fresh parsley, leaves and stems

So, what part of the chicken is actually a tender? Upon researching chicken sustainability, Serena discovered that this popular chicken cut is simply the small underside of the breast. That means one chicken has only two tenders, so a whole package of chicken tenders is from many birds. Armed with that knowledge, she decided to do a bit of home butchering and you can too—it's easy! Sharpen your knife and slice up your own tenders from two *whole* chicken breasts. Then, whip up this silky, briny, citrusy pan-sauced chicken, inspired by the classic Italian piccata dish.

Cut 1 lemon into ¼-inch slices and set aside. Using a Microplane or citrus zester, grate the zest from the other lemon over a large bowl. Cut the lemon in half and squeeze 1 tablespoon juice into a separate small bowl. Cut the remaining half into wedges for serving.

Add the cornmeal, flour, salt, and ¼ teaspoon pepper to the large bowl with the lemon zest and whisk to combine. Add half of the chicken strips and turn the pieces to evenly cover and coat the chicken.

Heat 2 tablespoons oil in a large skillet over medium-high heat. Add the breaded chicken and cook for 3 minutes, then flip the tenders and continue to cook until golden brown, an additional 2 to 3 minutes. Transfer to a serving platter to rest and let rise to an internal temperature of 165°F. Add the remaining 1 tablespoon oil to the skillet and repeat the coating, cooking, and resting with the second batch of chicken.

Add the wine to the hot skillet drippings and cook over medium heat, scraping up any browned bits, until the sauce is reduced by half, about 2 minutes. Add 1 cup water and the reserved lemon slices and bring to a boil. Cook until reduced by half, about 6 minutes. Remove from the heat, and stir in the reserved lemon juice, capers, parsley, and remaining ¼ teaspoon pepper.

To serve, pour the sauce over the chicken tenders on the platter and serve immediately with the reserved lemon wedges for squeezing.

Healthy Kitchen Hack: Our #1 eco-friendly chicken tip is: don't waste it. According to the USDA, raw chicken is extremely perishable and should be in the refrigerator for no more than 2 days. So, look to buying frozen chicken breasts (which usually cost less than fresh) or freeze fresh chicken immediately after purchase—but transfer it out of its original packaging to avoid freezer burn. To freeze without plastic, tightly wrap each piece of chicken in double or triple layers of waxed or butcher paper and secure with freezer tape. Heavy-duty aluminum foil can also be used, but make sure there are no tiny holes to allow in freezer burn.

Per Serving: Calories: 229; Total Fat: 10g; Saturated Fat: 2g; Cholesterol: 83mg; Sodium: 203mg; Total Carbohydrates: 6g; Fiber: 1g; Protein: 26g

"Making my own tenders seemed to allow for faster cook time. The lemon flavor was simply divine and the chicken was so tender. I felt like I was eating a meal prepared at a restaurant, but I was in my own house."

—Jessie from Glenwood, MD

North African Chicken Couscous Bowls

SERVES 6
Prep time: 15 minutes
Cook time: 25 minutes

Inspired by the staple tagine stews from Algiers, Morocco, and Tunisia, these super flavorful bowls are rich in traditional North African ingredients that are often associated with sweet recipes in North America and Europe, like cinnamon and dried fruit. Here we use chicken thighs, but feel free to use whatever meat or chicken you have on hand. Or go vegetarian and swap in two cans of chickpeas for the chicken. Adjust the seasoning to your preferred level of heat, spice, and sweetness with the ideas in our Healthy Kitchen Hack.

1 teaspoon ground cumin

½ teaspoon ground cinnamon

½ teaspoon ground turmeric

½ teaspoon kosher or sea salt, divided

¼ teaspoon black pepper

⅛ teaspoon cayenne pepper or crushed red pepper

1½ pounds skinless, boneless chicken thighs, cut into 1½-inch pieces

1 large onion (any type), cut into 1-inch wedges

3 tablespoons extra-virgin olive oil

3 garlic cloves, minced

¾ cup dried figs or prunes, coarsely chopped

3 tablespoons tomato paste

4 cups Veggie Scraps Broth (page 120) or low-sodium vegetable broth, divided

1 lemon

4 scallions (green onions), green and white parts, thinly sliced
Save the stems!
See page 70

1½ cups uncooked regular or whole-wheat couscous

In a large bowl, mix together the cumin, cinnamon, turmeric, ¼ teaspoon salt, black pepper, and cayenne pepper. Pour out half of the mixture into a small bowl and set aside. Add the chicken and onion to the large bowl and toss with your hands until everything is well coated. Set aside.

In a large stockpot or Dutch oven, heat the oil over medium heat. Add the garlic and the reserved spice mix. Cook for 30 seconds, stirring constantly. Add the seasoned chicken and onion and cook for 5 minutes, stirring frequently, until the onion starts to soften. Stir in the figs and tomato paste. Add 1¾ cups broth, turn the heat to medium-high, and bring to a boil. Reduce the heat to medium-low and simmer for 15 minutes, stirring occasionally—the stew will start to thicken slightly. Remove from the heat. Using a Microplane or citrus zester, grate the zest from the lemon over the pot, then cut the lemon in half and squeeze in the juice through a strainer. Mix into the stew.

While the chicken cooks, make the couscous. In a medium saucepan, bring the remaining 2¼ cups broth and the scallions to a boil. Remove from the heat, stir in the couscous, and cover. Let sit for 5 minutes then add the remaining ¼ teaspoon salt and fluff well with a fork.

To serve, divide the couscous into six bowls and spoon the chicken stew with its sauce on top.

Healthy Kitchen Hack: For extra spicy heat, slice up a jalapeño pepper and add it with the figs and tomato paste. For smokier heat, add ½ teaspoon smoked paprika to the spice mix. For more sweetness, increase the dried figs or prunes to 1 cup or whisk in 1 tablespoon honey when simmering.

Per Serving: **Calories: 351; Total Fat: 9g; Saturated Fat: 2g; Cholesterol: 35mg; Sodium: 297mg; Total Carbohydrates: 53g; Fiber: 6g; Protein: 15g**

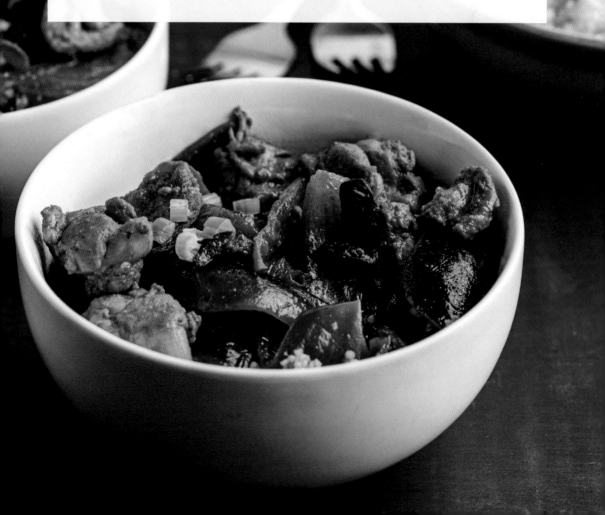

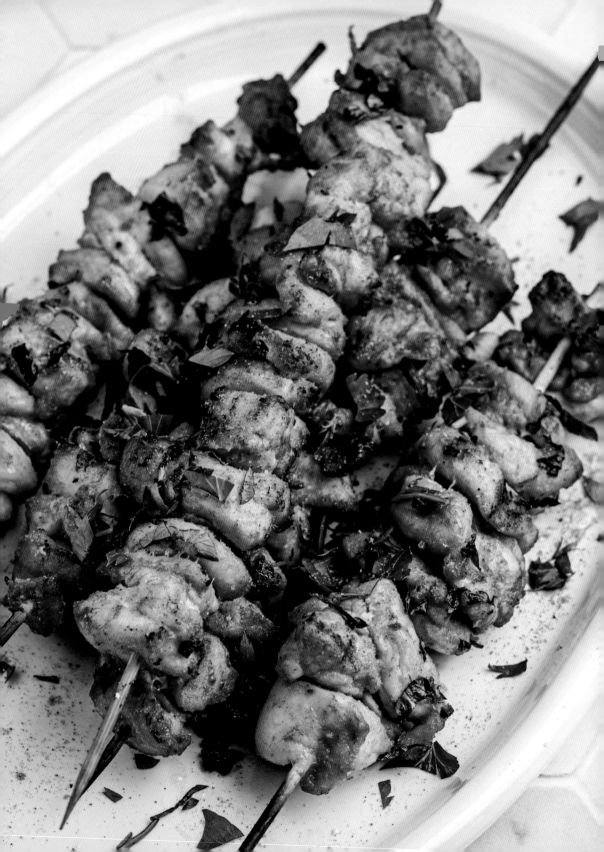

Harissa-Spiced Chicken Kebabs

SERVES 4
Prep time: 15 minutes
Cook time: 15 minutes

1 lime

2 tablespoons sweet paprika

1 tablespoon ground cumin

1 teaspoon ground coriander

½ teaspoon smoked paprika

½ teaspoon garlic powder

½ teaspoon kosher or sea salt

½ teaspoon black pepper

3 tablespoons extra-virgin olive oil

1 medium onion (any type), cut into 8 wedges (without removing the root end so they remain intact)

1½ pounds boneless, skinless chicken thighs, cut into 1-inch pieces

1 cup chopped fresh mint or cilantro, leaves and stems

2 large whole-wheat pita breads, halved crosswise and toasted (optional)

We develop our recipes to be as easy as possible for home cooks everywhere. So when it comes to including a "specialty" ingredient in a dish, we have a test: can Serena find it in the regular grocery store in her mid-sized Midwestern town? Alas, harissa, the peppery and smoky reddish pepper paste originally from Tunisia, hasn't made it to Edwardsville, Illinois . . . yet. We're sure it won't be long before this intoxicating Middle Eastern condiment, commonly used as a dip or marinade or to add flavor to other dishes, becomes popular from coast to coast. But for now, Serena did the next best thing and came up with a somewhat exotic-tasting spice blend that mimics harissa but is created from easy-to-find spices—so you can enjoy these authentic North African flavors wherever you live. But if you're lucky enough to find harissa, you can substitute ¼ cup for all the spices and the oil here.

Using a Microplane or citrus zester, grate the zest from the lime over a large bowl, then cut the lime in half and squeeze in the juice. Add the sweet paprika, cumin, coriander, smoked paprika, garlic powder, salt, pepper, and oil and whisk to combine. Add the onion wedges and carefully toss to coat, keeping the wedges intact. Transfer the onions to a plate and brush any extra spice paste back into the bowl. Add the chicken to the spice paste and toss to coat. Cover with a plate and marinate at room temperature for 20 minutes. (If making ahead, chill up to 12 hours in the refrigerator. Set out at room temperature for 30 minutes before grilling.)

Thread the chicken onto four to six (10-inch or longer) metal skewers (or wooden skewers that can be composted), keeping the chunks close together so the meat stays juicy.

Coat the cold grill with cooking spray, then heat to 400°F, or medium-high heat. Place the skewers and the onions, round edges down, on the hot grill over direct heat. Cook the skewers, turning every 2 to 3 minutes, until the chicken is cooked through and just barely

continued

charred, about 15 minutes. Remove the skewers from the grill and let rest for at least 5 minutes to allow the juices to set. Do not turn the onions as they cook; remove when lightly charred, about 18 minutes.

Transfer the chicken and onions to a serving platter. Sprinkle with the mint and serve as is or stuffed inside pita bread halves, if you like.

Healthy Kitchen Hack: Take your homemade harissa paste to the next level by using whole spices (available in regular supermarkets) that you toast and grind yourself. In a dry skillet over medium heat, heat 1 tablespoon cumin seeds, 1 teaspoon whole coriander, and ½ teaspoon whole black peppercorns for 3 to 4 minutes until fragrant, shaking occasionally. Grind the toasted spices with a mortar and pestle or a spice grinder. Add to the paprika, garlic powder, salt, lime zest, lime juice, and oil as described above. Besides chicken, use this vibrant spice paste to flavor grilled veggies like corn on the cob (or as we do with our Roasted Harissa Zucchini Spears on page 98), mix into couscous, fold into scrambled eggs, spread over fish, or use as a condiment swap anywhere you typically use hot sauce. Store in the refrigerator for up to a month.

Per Serving (chicken and onions): Calories: 332; Total Fat: 18g; Saturated Fat: 3.5g; Cholesterol: 160mg; Sodium: 409mg; Total Carbohydrates: 7g; Fiber: 2g; Protein: 34g

Creamy Chicken Skillet Supper with Greens

SERVES 6
Prep time: 10 minutes
Cook time: 25 minutes

1 (2-ounce) tin anchovies in olive oil, undrained

2½ tablespoons extra-virgin olive oil, divided

2 garlic cloves, minced

1½ pounds boneless, skinless chicken breasts, cut into 1-inch pieces

½ teaspoon kosher or sea salt, divided

½ teaspoon black pepper, divided

3 scallions (green onions), green and white parts, thinly sliced
*Save the stems!
See page 70*

8 cups (12 ounces) chopped fresh spinach

1 cup chopped parsley and/or cilantro, leaves and stems

1 cup plain 2% Greek yogurt

Deanna's favorite Zesty Garlic Sauce (page 100) shows up again in this super easy, one-pan chicken dinner that's loaded with protein, vitamins, minerals, and (most importantly) sublime savory flavor. Spinach is the featured green because we love how fast it cooks, but this recipe will also work to use up any green veggies that are lurking in your fridge (see this recipe's Healthy Kitchen Hack). Enjoy it right out of the skillet, over pasta or couscous, or with pita bread to sop up every saucy bite.

Using a fork, remove the anchovies from the tin and set aside.

In a large skillet, heat 2 tablespoons olive oil and all the oil from the anchovy tin over medium heat. Add the garlic and cook, stirring constantly, for about 30 seconds. Reduce the heat to medium-low, add 6 anchovies (save the remaining anchovies for another use) and mash them up with the back of a wooden spoon or spatula as you stir frequently for 1 minute. Continue to cook, stirring occasionally, for 10 more minutes, until the anchovies are completely incorporated into the oil. Remove the pan from the stove and pour the contents into a small bowl. Set aside to cool.

Return the skillet to the stove and heat the remaining ½ tablespoon oil over medium heat. Sprinkle the chicken with ¼ teaspoon each salt and pepper. Add the chicken and scallions and cook, stirring frequently, for 5 minutes. Add half of the spinach, stir, and cook for 2 minutes until partially wilted, then add the remaining spinach. Stir and cook until the chicken is cooked through and the spinach is completely wilted, an additional 2 to 3 minutes. Remove from the heat. Using a lid to keep the chicken and spinach in the skillet, carefully tilt the skillet into a measuring cup and drain off most of the liquid, leaving about 1 tablespoon in the skillet. (Or if you find this too tricky to do, slightly tilt the skillet and remove most of

continued

the liquid by spoonfuls into the measuring cup.) Stir the parsley and remaining ¼ teaspoon each salt and pepper into the chicken mixture. Set aside.

Add the yogurt to the bowl with the anchovy garlic oil. Add 2 tablespoons of the skillet liquid from the measuring cup and whisk. Add the yogurt sauce to the skillet with the chicken and fold all the ingredients together. If the sauce seems too thick, stir in more of the skillet liquid, 1 tablespoon at a time.

Healthy Kitchen Hack: Switch up the greens in this recipe using whatever leafies you have on hand. More delicate greens like arugula, watercress, and Swiss chard can be swapped for the spinach. If you have hardy ones like chopped collards, kale, or mustard greens, add them to the skillet at the start with the chicken and scallions since they take longer to cook.

Per Serving: Calories: 278; Total Fat: 15g; Saturated Fat: 3g; Cholesterol: 91mg; Sodium: 435mg; Total Carbohydrates: 4g; Fiber: 1g; Protein: 32g

Spring Chicken with Barley, Carrots, and Artichokes

SERVES 6
Prep time: 20 minutes
Cook time: 60 to 90 minutes

2 (14-ounce) cans large whole artichoke hearts (not marinated), drained (liquid saved for another use)

3 tablespoons extra-virgin olive oil, divided

¾ teaspoon kosher or sea salt, divided

2 pounds carrots, unpeeled, cut in 1-inch slices

1 lemon

1 garlic clove, finely chopped

1 tablespoon dried oregano

¼ teaspoon black pepper

1 (4- to 5-pound) roasting chicken (neck and giblets removed and reserved for another use, see Hack)

2 cups quick pearl barley (see Note)

¼ cup chopped fresh chives

We know some people (Deanna) can be intimidated by cooking a whole bird, but it's actually easy, economical, and yes, eco-friendly (chickens only have two breasts, after all, so buying a whole package of breasts means someone needs to find a use for the rest of those parts!). While this recipe takes about 1½ hours, most of that is oven time *and* you will be making your entire meal all together in one pan (OK—two sheet pans!)—with perhaps even some leftovers to spare. So, prepare your family to feast on crispy oven-fried artichokes, hearty and schmaltz-rich carrot and barley stuffing, and tender succulent chicken.

Arrange the oven racks to the upper-middle and lower-middle positions. Line two large rimmed baking sheets with aluminum foil and place one sheet on the lower rack in the oven. Preheat the oven to 400°F (with the sheet inside). Coat the foil on the second pan with cooking spray; set aside.

Cut the artichokes in half, transfer to a clean tea towel, and pat dry. In a large bowl, gently toss together the artichokes, 4 teaspoons oil, and ¼ teaspoon salt. On the cooking spray–coated baking sheet, arrange some of the artichokes cut-side up and some cut-side down. Set aside.

To the same large bowl, add the carrots and 1 teaspoon oil; toss to combine. Set aside.

Using a Microplane or citrus zester, grate the zest from the lemon into a medium bowl. (Save the remaining lemon for the barley.) Whisk in the remaining 4 teaspoons oil, garlic, oregano, remaining ½ teaspoon salt, and pepper.

Place the chicken breast-side up in a 9 × 13-inch pan to contain the juices while you season it. If the chicken came with a giblet bag and/or the chicken neck stuffed inside the cavity, remove it (see the Healthy Kitchen Hack on how to use giblets). Starting

continued

at the open end of the carcass, loosen the skin from the chicken breast and meaty part of the thighs and drumsticks by inserting your fingers and gently pushing between the skin and meat. Rub the oregano mixture under the loosened chicken skin.

Using oven mitts, carefully remove the preheated baking sheet from the oven, coat the foil with cooking spray, and immediately place the chicken, breast-side up, on the sheet. Arrange the carrots around the chicken. Put the sheet on the lower rack in the oven and the artichokes on the top rack. Bake the artichokes for 50 minutes or until they are turning brown on the bottoms and edges. When you remove the artichokes from the oven, stir the carrots and rotate the chicken pan (on the same oven rack). Bake the chicken for an additional 10 to 40 minutes for a total of 60 to 90 minutes (depending on chicken size) or until a meat thermometer inserted into the meaty part of the thigh reads 165°F. The carrots will be done after about 1 hour, and so will a 4-pound chicken; if your chicken is larger, you can remove the carrots before the chicken is completely done, although we also like them cooked longer to a deep mahogany brown color with a larger chicken.

While the chicken cooks, make the barley on the stove according to the package directions, without salt. When the barley is done, cut the reserved lemon in half and squeeze in the juice. Cover to keep warm.

Slide the cooked artichokes off the aluminum foil and back onto the baking sheet; save the foil.

When the chicken is done, use tongs and a large metal spatula to transfer it to a cutting board and tent loosely with the saved foil; let rest for at least 10 minutes. Turn off the oven. Scrape the carrots and chicken drippings from the baking sheet into the barley and stir; cover to keep warm and to allow the drippings to flavor the barley while the chicken rests. Return the artichokes to the warm (but turned-off) oven to crisp up for an additional 5 to 10 minutes (they are especially crispy when hot out of the oven!).

Carve the chicken into serving pieces. To serve, spoon the carrot-barley stuffing onto a serving platter and top with the chicken pieces and the crispy artichokes. Sprinkle with the chives.

Note: Pearl barley has the bran partially removed, resulting in quicker cooking times; we use "quick" barley, which cooks in 10 minutes and for which 1 serving is ⅓ cup. If you have a different pearl barley, make enough for 6 servings and adjust the cooking time per the package instructions.

Healthy Kitchen Hack: When you buy a whole chicken, giblets—the liver, heart, and gizzard—and sometimes the neck are often in a paper or plastic bag stuffed inside the bird. They can be a treat, especially if you embrace the goal of using every consumable part of your chicken—but knowing how to make them tasty can be a challenge! To begin, make a rich chicken broth. Combine the giblets, except the liver, in a saucepan along with chopped celery, chopped onion, and enough lightly salted water to cover, and some herbs if desired. Bring to a boil (skimming off the foam if desired), then cover and simmer until tender, about 1 hour. Add the liver and simmer until tender, an additional 5 to 10 minutes. Remove the giblets and finely chop; discard the neck bones (the meat will have fallen off into the broth). Strain the broth and store in the refrigerator or freezer to use in any recipe calling for chicken broth. Add the chopped giblets to casseroles, stuffings, or baked pasta dishes, or make a sandwich filling by stirring them into our Olive Oil and Yogurt spread (page 233). And don't toss that chicken carcass! Follow the instructions above using the carcass instead of or in addition to the giblets to make more chicken broth (it freezes beautifully).

Per Serving (chicken, barley, and vegetables): **Calories: 560; Total Fat: 19g; Saturated Fat: 4g; Cholesterol: 103mg; Sodium: 630mg; Total Carbohydrates: 55g; Fiber: 12g; Protein: 42g**

"While this isn't a quick 20-minute recipe, after you put the ingredients on the sheet pans, the oven does the rest of the work! This is a great meal and we loved having lots of leftovers."

—Bonnie from Lakewood, CO

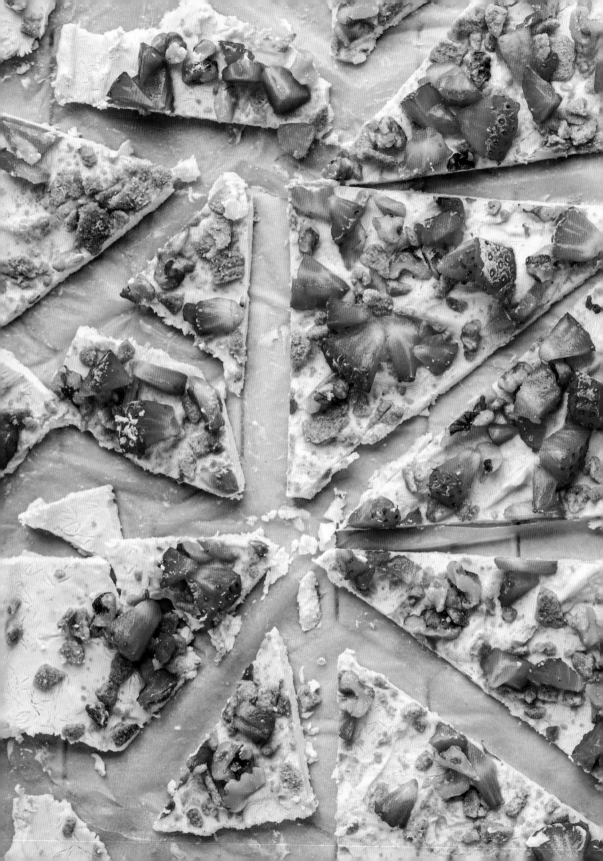

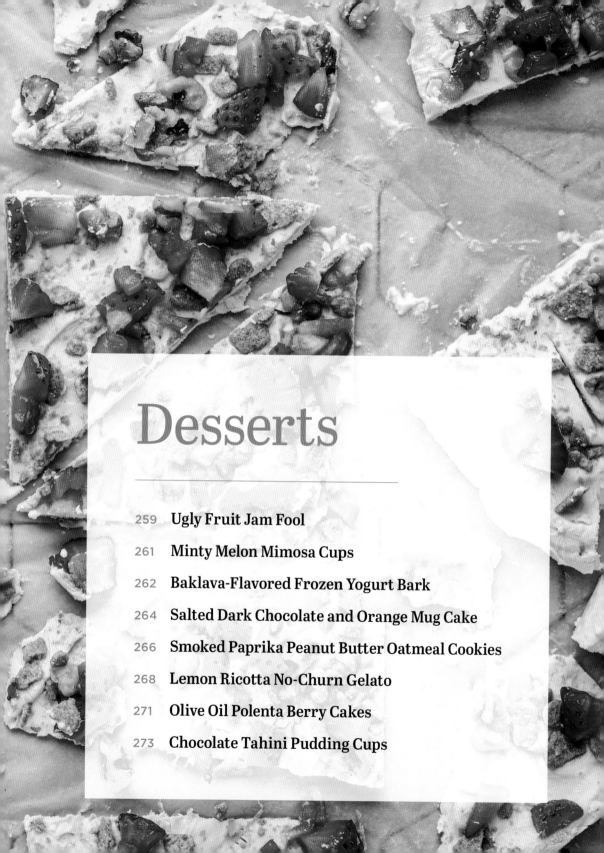

Desserts

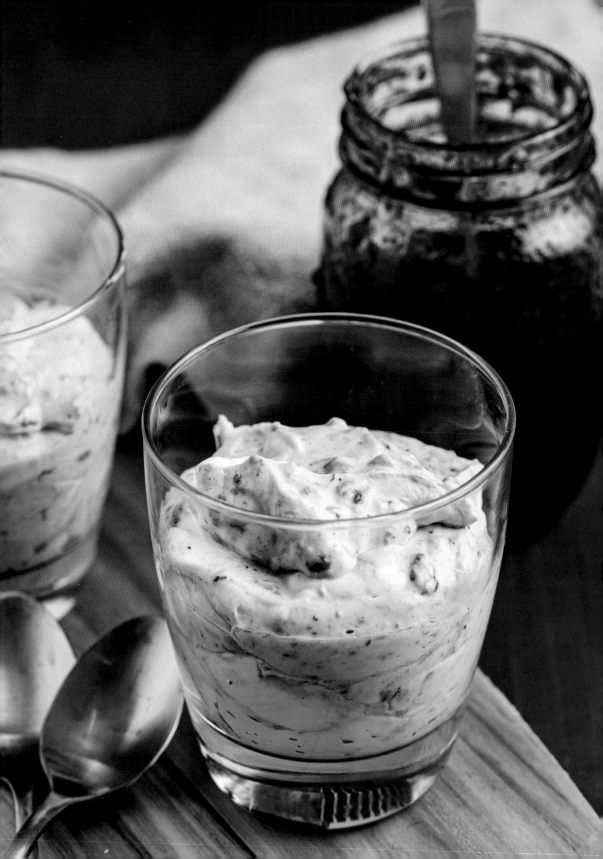

Ugly Fruit Jam Fool

SERVES 6
Prep time: 5 minutes,
 plus 2 hours resting and
 cooling time
Cook time: 20 minutes

1 lemon

4 cups chopped very
ripe or overripe fruit

⅓ cup plus
2 tablespoons honey,
divided

1 cup heavy cream

1 cup plain 2% Greek
yogurt

2 teaspoons vanilla
extract

It all began one late summer morning when Serena's daughter's lunch box left for school with a beautiful hand-picked local peach . . . and then returned home with a sad squishy peach no one wanted. Ugly Fruit Jam was born. Now, any less-than-desirable or overripe fruits at the Ball household—such as peaches, plums, grapes, mangoes, pears, apples, berries, even tomatoes!—are chopped, sweetened, and microwaved into a spreadable topping. The jam becomes the topping we use in this dreamy dessert known as a fruit fool, which is cooked fruit folded into mounds of whipped cream or custard. After whipping up this oh-so-easy dessert, you'll still have plenty of leftover jam to top pancakes, our Olive Oil Polenta Berry Cakes (page 271), or our favorite Mediterranean version of the PB&J: tahini and jam sandwiches!

Using a Microplane or citrus zester, grate the zest from the lemon over a large (at least 2-quart) glass bowl; cut the lemon in half and squeeze in 2 tablespoons juice. (Save the remaining lemon for another use.) Add the fruit and ⅓ cup honey and mash with a potato masher or fork until the fruit reaches the texture you prefer. Set aside at room temperature for at least 30 minutes or more depending on the fruit (30 minutes for berries, 45 minutes for stone fruit, and 1 hour for apples and pears).

Microwave the bowl of fruit, uncovered, on high power for 5 minutes. Using oven mitts, remove the bowl and stir well. Microwave for another 5 minutes, then stir. Continue to microwave in 2-minute increments, stirring after each, until the fruit begins to thicken, for about an additional 6 minutes. The jam is ready when the juices are rapidly bubbling and it is a fairly thick but still runny syrup consistency (it will *not* be a solid jam consistency yet), 15 to 16 minutes total microwave time. Chill in the refrigerator for at least an hour. The jam will continue to thicken quite a bit while cooling in the refrigerator, so do not overcook or the honey will crystallize (but if this

continued

happens, add 1 to 2 tablespoons water and microwave at lower power).
See more jam-making tips in this recipe's Healthy Kitchen Hack.

After chilling, check the jam's consistency, and if you want thicker
jam, simply microwave it again to the desired thickness. The recipe
makes about 2½ cups of jam. Store in (reused) half-pint jam or mason
jars in the fridge for up to 2 weeks or freeze for up to 4 months.

To make the fool, whip the cream in a large bowl with an electric
mixer or in a stand mixer until soft peaks form. Add the yogurt and
vanilla; turn on the mixer and drizzle in the remaining 2 tablespoons
honey. Whip until firm peaks form (the peaks hold when the beaters are
lifted). Transfer to a serving bowl and spoon in ¾ cup jam. Using a spoon
or a spatula, gently swirl the jam through the whipped cream without
completely incorporating. To serve, spoon into six dessert cups.

Healthy Kitchen Hack: For jam-making success, follow these tips:
Start with fruit that is super ripe and/or almost mushy. Use at least
2 tablespoons lemon juice because its natural pectin will help thicken
the jam. Let the fruit sit in the honey and lemon juice for a minimum
of 30 minutes; this maceration process helps draw the juice out of
the fruit and will allow for the juice to more easily evaporate during
cooking, concentrating the fruit sugars for better-tasting jam. For fruits
like apples, pears, and peaches, there is no need to remove the skin as
it adds flavor and fiber. If you want a smoother jam, puree part or all
of the finished jam using an immersion blender or a regular blender.
Lastly, mix it up if there are several types of overripe fruit on your
counter; Serena once made a killer peach-mango-tomato jam!

Per Serving: Calories: 216; Total Fat: 15g; Saturated Fat: 9g; Cholesterol: 49mg;
Sodium: 23mg; Total Carbohydrates: 16g; Fiber: 1g; Protein: 5g

"I made this jam with strawberries and it was so
good, I started eating it with a spoon before even
making the rest of this recipe!"

—Sally from Columbus, OH

Minty Melon Mimosa Cups

SERVES 6
Prep time: 10 minutes

2 navel oranges

2 (3½- to 4-pound) melons, rind removed and flesh cut into cubes (about 7 cups)
Save the seeds! See the Hack

2 tablespoons honey

½ teaspoon ground ginger

⅛ teaspoon kosher or sea salt

1½ cups prosecco, sparkling rosé, or blood orange Italian soda

¼ cup chopped fresh mint or basil, leaves and stems

We're crushing on this sparkling and easy upgrade to your usual fruit cup. Enjoy this recipe during peak melon season, which is typically May through November for cantaloupe, honeydew, and other varieties. In super hot weather, freeze your cut melon ahead of time for a few hours for the perfect meal finale to a summer day. Portion it out in pretty glasses and serve with a spoon *and* a (reusable) straw!

Using a Microplane or citrus zester, grate the zest from the oranges over a large bowl; cut the oranges in half and squeeze in all the juice. Add the cubed melon, honey, ginger, and salt and mix well. (At this point, you can refrigerate the flavored melon for up to 24 hours.)

When ready to serve, gently stir in the prosecco and mint. Portion into wine or drinking glasses and serve righ away.

Healthy Kitchen Hack: Roast those melon seeds! Deanna was just as surprised as you may be to discover that melon seeds are edible and pretty yummy when roasted much like squash seeds. Follow our oven method on page 61, but check after only 5 minutes as melon seeds are much smaller than squash seeds.

Per Serving: Calories: 152; Total Fat: 0g; Saturated Fat: 0g; Cholesterol: 0mg; Sodium: 79mg; Total Carbohydrates: 27g; Fiber: 2g; Protein: 1g

Baklava-Flavored Frozen Yogurt Bark

SERVES 6
Prep time: 10 minutes
Chill time: 2 to 3 hours

2 cups plain whole-milk Greek yogurt

2 tablespoons plus 1 teaspoon honey, divided

1 teaspoon vanilla extract *or* ¼ teaspoon almond extract

1 lemon

½ cup crumbled whole-grain crackers and/or breakfast cereal

¼ cup chopped walnuts or other nuts

½ cup frozen or fresh fruit, such as chopped peaches or strawberries, or whole blueberries

It's a happy day in the Ball household when their neighbor Janice shows up with a large tray of homemade baklava, the buttery Greek phyllo dough dessert, traditionally layered with chopped walnuts and honey. Inspired by these main flavors, Serena created this super easy dessert to whip up any day. Feel free to customize by swapping in whatever nuts, crackers, cereal, and/or fruit you have on hand.

Spread a sheet of parchment paper on a large rimmed baking sheet; clear a flat area in your freezer for the baking sheet.

In a large bowl, whisk together the yogurt, 2 tablespoons honey, and vanilla extract. Spread evenly on the prepared baking sheet, to about ⅛-inch thickness.

Using a Microplane or citrus zester, grate the zest from the lemon evenly over the yogurt (save the remaining lemon for another use). Drizzle the remaining 1 teaspoon honey over the yogurt. Using a silicone scraper, make one or two swirls through the yogurt to incorporate the zest and honey. Evenly sprinkle the crackers, nuts, and fruit over the yogurt. Freeze for 2 to 3 hours until frozen firm.

Cut or break the bark into pieces, remove the parchment paper, and serve immediately. Alternatively, freeze the bark pieces in a freezer-friendly container for up to 3 months.

Healthy Kitchen Hack: This recipe is an easy and yummy way to use up those last couple of broken whole-grain crackers or breakfast cereal crumbs at the bottom of the box. Or, stir those last bits into a bowl of oatmeal or other hot whole-grain. Another use is to swap them for bread crumbs to top a casserole or to mix them into a coating for baked fish sticks.

Per Serving: Calories: 170; Total Fat: 8g; Saturated Fat: 3g; Cholesterol: 12mg; Sodium: 58mg; Total Carbohydrates: 15g; Fiber: 1g; Protein: 10g

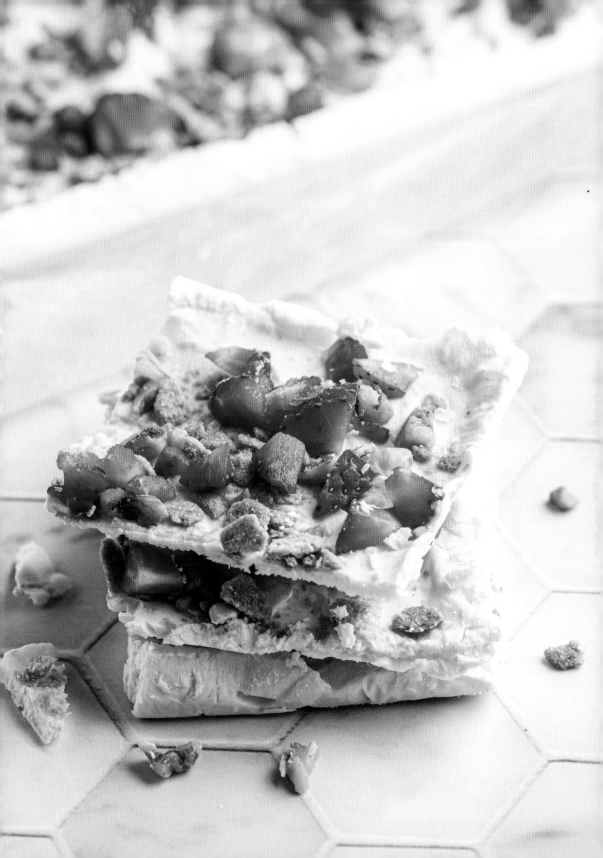

Salted Dark Chocolate and Orange Mug Cake

SERVES 1
Prep time: 5 minutes
Cook time: 1 minute

2 teaspoons extra-virgin olive oil

2 clementines, *or* 1 mandarin, *or* 1 navel orange

2 teaspoons honey

½ teaspoon vanilla extract

2 tablespoons white whole-wheat flour, whole-wheat flour, or all-purpose flour

2 teaspoons unsweetened cocoa powder

¼ teaspoon baking powder

2 pinches kosher or sea salt, divided

1 tablespoon dark chocolate chips

Have your cake (ready in just 6 minutes) and eat it too. Since you can whip up this personal-size chocolatey citrus cake with Mediterranean staples that you probably already have in your pantry, there's no "running to the store for just a few things." Because if you're like us, that often results in buying extra items that we don't really need, instead of using up what we already have on hand. With that in mind, if you don't have a fresh orange, swap in 2 tablespoons of store-bought orange juice or other fruit juice.

Pour the oil into a coffee cup, 6-ounce ramekin, or other small microwave-safe bowl; swirl to coat the bottom with oil. Using a Microplane or citrus zester, grate the zest from the orange into the cup until you have about ¼ teaspoon zest. Cut the orange in half and squeeze in 2 tablespoons juice; if you can't squeeze out quite 2 tablespoons, use water to make up the difference. (Enjoy the remaining orange as a snack or toss it into our Creamy Cantaloupe-Orange Smoothie on page 27.) Add the honey and vanilla and mix well.

In a small bowl, mix together the flour, cocoa powder, baking soda, and a good pinch of salt. Add to the wet ingredients in the mug and stir well until there are no dry spots. Sprinkle in the chocolate chips.

Microwave on high power for 30 seconds. If the center has more than a ½-inch circle that is not set, microwave for 5 to 10 seconds more. Sprinkle with the remaining pinch of salt. Cool for 5 minutes before enjoying.

Healthy Kitchen Hack: One of our tricks to using less added sugar in baked goods is to use a sprinkle of salt. Our mug cake only contains 2 teaspoons of honey (plus chocolate chips) compared to typical mug cake recipes, which tend to have at least double that amount of added sugar. When your tongue tastes a combination of salt and sweet, the sweetness seems more intense, so you can often cut back on the added sugar. So, the next time you bake a batch of cookies, brownies, or bars, plan on adding a sprinkle of kosher or sea salt (the larger salt crystals taste more pronounced) to the tops. Then try cutting out at least a couple tablespoons of sugar from the original recipe.

Per Serving: Calories: 277; Total Fat: 15g; Saturated Fat: 4g; Cholesterol: 0mg; Sodium: 243mg; Total Carbohydrates: 37g; Fiber: 4g; Protein: 4g

Smoked Paprika Peanut Butter Oatmeal Cookies

MAKES 28 COOKIES
Prep time: 15 minutes
Cook time: 10 minutes

1 cup peanut butter

½ cup honey

3 tablespoons extra-virgin olive oil

1 large egg

1 teaspoon vanilla extract

2½ cups gluten-free old-fashioned rolled oats, divided

1 teaspoon ground cinnamon

½ teaspoon smoked paprika

½ teaspoon baking soda

¼ teaspoon kosher or sea salt

"These cookies are really yummy with a fun texture that reminds me of no-bake cookies. I loved the spice combo, too."

—**Kristell from Billings, MT**

Here's our peanut butter cookie and oatmeal cookie mash-up with a Mediterranean spice twist! Soft and chewy centers with a slight crunch plus a hint of smoke make these treats something special. But if you're not feeling spicy, you can swap in another pantry ingredient for the smoked paprika, such as grated nutmeg, sesame seeds, cocoa powder, instant espresso powder, ground cardamom—the list goes on!

Arrange the oven racks to the upper-middle and lower-middle positions. Preheat the oven to 350°F.

In a large mixing bowl with an electric mixer or a stand mixer fitted with the paddle attachment, mix the peanut butter and honey until well blended. Add the oil, egg, and vanilla and mix until all ingredients are incorporated.

In a food processor or blender, pulse/blend 1 cup oats until they resemble a coarse flour. Dump the oat flour into the bowl with the peanut butter–honey mixture, along with the remaining 1½ cups oats, cinnamon, smoked paprika, baking soda, and salt. Mix until all the dry ingredients are well incorporated.

Measure the dough into 1½-tablespoon portions and roll into balls. Spread out onto two ungreased baking sheets. Using a fork to flatten the cookie, press down once and then another time perpendicularly to make a crisscross pattern on top. (If the fork starts to get sticky, wet it with cool water between each pattern press.) Bake for 10 to 12 minutes, until the cookies slightly puff up and just begin to brown around the edges; the cookies will not look fully baked. Or, if you like extra crispy cookies, add 2 more minutes to the baking time. Remove from the oven, leave the cookies on the pans for 5 minutes, and then transfer to wire racks to cool completely.

Healthy Kitchen Hack: We try to bake our desserts and treats right after or before we're using the oven for a main dish or meal. This way, it's already preheated and

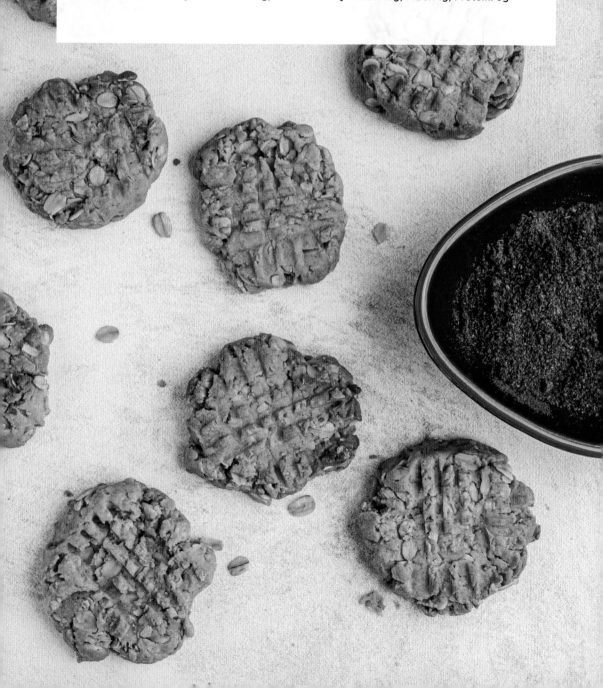

will be ready to use for the next recipe immediately. It saves energy and time in the kitchen—win-win!

Lemon Ricotta No-Churn Gelato

SERVES 8

Prep time: 10 minutes
Chill time: 3 to 4 hours

2 lemons

½ cup honey

⅛ teaspoon kosher or sea salt

2 batches Made-in-Minutes Homemade Ricotta Cheese recipe (page 48) *or* 1½ cups store-bought whole-milk ricotta cheese

1 cup whole milk

½ cup heavy cream

No, you don't need a fancy ice cream maker to whip up a batch of homemade gelato. If you have a freezer, a few staple ingredients, and chill time, you're equipped to serve up delectable Mediterranean-inspired ice cream with ease— and no packaging to recycle, either! Traditionally, gelato contains more milk than cream, which allows the intense flavors to shine through. The tangy, bright lemon essence and the slightly sweet, creamy, dreamy ricotta makes this gelato something special. But we also want you to think of this recipe as a starting point to get innovative with different mix-ins to create your own special gelato flavor! See this recipe's Healthy Kitchen Hack for ideas.

Using a Microplane or citrus zester, grate the zest from the lemons over a large mixing bowl or a stand mixer bowl (you should get 3 to 4 teaspoons). Cut the lemons in half and squeeze in the juice through a strainer, measuring out 4 to 5 tablespoons. (Save any extra lemon juice for another use). Add the honey and salt. Mix with electric beaters, a whisk, or the stand mixer whisk attachment until the salt dissolves, about 1 minute.

Spoon the ricotta cheese into the mixing bowl, then add the milk and cream. Mix/whisk again until you have a creamy and nearly smooth liquid, for 4 to 5 minutes.

Pour the gelato mix into an 8- or 9-inch square baking pan. Freeze for 3 hours for a soft-serve consistency or 4 hours or more for a firmer gelato. While the gelato will be at its creamiest texture at 3 to 4 hours after freezing, if you are not ready to serve it, transfer it to a sealable freezer container and store in the freezer for up to 3 weeks. Let it sit at room temperature for 10 to 15 minutes to soften a bit and make it easier to scoop.

Healthy Kitchen Hack: Create a rainbow of different types of "sustainable" gelato flavors by adding mix-ins to this lemon recipe! Use up your fresh fruit that's approaching the overripe stage. Finely chop softened stone fruit like peaches, plums, cherries, or apricots or mash up those tired-looking blackberries, raspberries, strawberries, or blueberries. Mix in up to 1 cup fruit as the last step before freezing. Or mince and mix in 2 to 3 tablespoons of whatever fresh herbs you might have lurking in the fridge like mint, basil, or thyme.

Per Serving: Calories: 192; Total Fat: 10g; Saturated Fat: 6g; Cholesterol: 35mg; Sodium: 91mg; Total Carbohydrates: 21g; Fiber: 0g; Protein: 7g

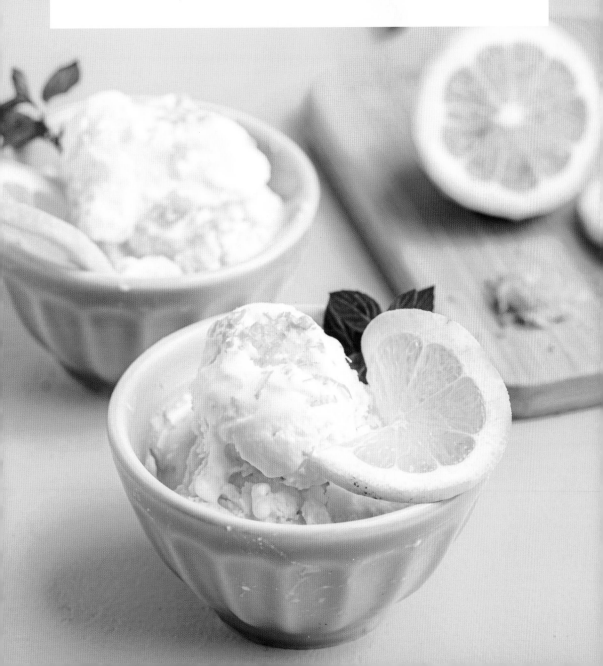

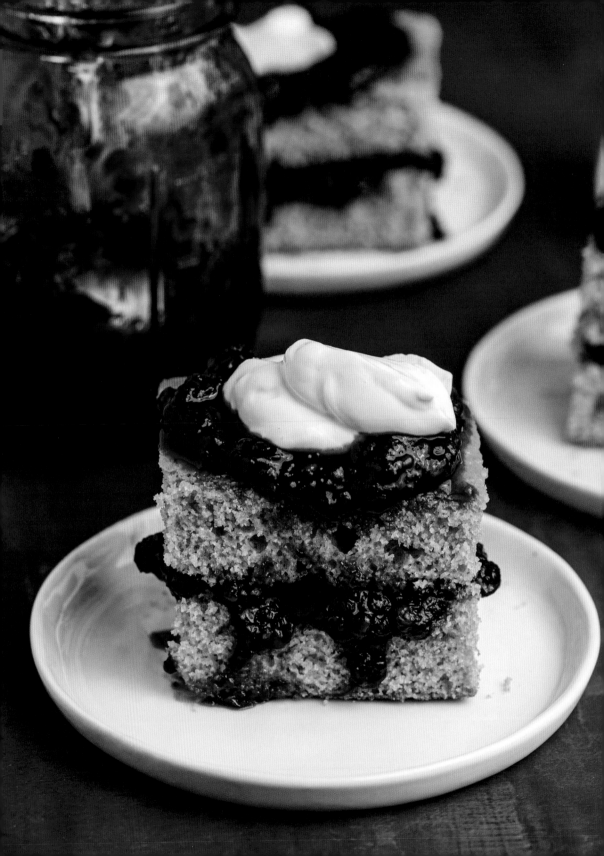

Olive Oil Polenta Berry Cakes

SERVES 12
Prep time: 10 minutes
Cook time: 20 minutes

1 cup cornmeal

¾ cup all-purpose flour

½ cup whole-wheat pastry flour, white whole-wheat flour, or whole-wheat flour

2 teaspoons baking powder

½ teaspoon baking soda

¼ teaspoon kosher or sea salt

1 lemon

1 cup buttermilk or plain kefir

⅓ cup honey

¼ cup extra-virgin olive oil

2 large eggs

1 batch Ugly Fruit Jam (page 259), or 1 (20-ounce) bag frozen mixed berries, thawed, or 4 cups mixed fresh raspberries, blueberries, blackberries, and/ or sliced strawberries (see Note)

1 tablespoon sugar (optional; see Note)

1½ cups vanilla or lemon 2% Greek yogurt

Fresh mint or basil leaves (optional)

Here's our Italian twist on the all-American classic strawberry shortcake. Instead of a biscuit-like base, we use nutrient-rich cornmeal—in addition to flour—to create a moist and slightly dense cake with an appealing toasted corn flavor. While berries are the traditional fruit topping of choice, you can swap in just about any type of fresh fruit that might not be looking its best on your counter or in your fridge via our Ugly Fruit Jam recipe (page 259). Top it off with a dollop of cool and creamy vanilla yogurt with some fresh mint or basil, if you have it on hand.

Preheat the oven to 425°F. Coat an 8- or 9-inch square baking pan with cooking spray.

In a large bowl, whisk together the cornmeal, flours, baking powder, baking soda, and salt; set aside.

Using a Microplane or citrus zester, grate the zest from the lemon over a medium bowl; cut the lemon in half and squeeze in the juice. Add the buttermilk, honey, oil, and eggs and whisk until all the ingredients are incorporated.

Pour the wet ingredients into the bowl with the dry ingredients and mix until just incorporated. Pour the batter into the prepared pan and use a spatula to spread it until evenly distributed. Bake for 18 to 22 minutes, until the cornbread starts to turn golden brown around the edges and a toothpick inserted in the center comes out clean. Remove from the oven and cool on a wire rack for about 10 minutes.

Cut the cornbread into 12 rectangular pieces. To serve, cut a shortcake in half lengthwise and place one half on a plate. Spoon about 1 tablespoon jam (or 2 tablespoons thawed or fresh fruit) onto the bottom half. Top with the other shortcake half. Spoon an additional 2 teaspoons jam (or 2 tablespoons thawed or fresh fruit) on top. Top with 2 tablespoons yogurt and fresh mint if desired. Serve immediately.

Note: If you're using frozen mixed berries instead of the Ugly Fruit Jam, empty the berries into a bowl to let them thaw while you're making the shortcakes. When the fruit

continued

is partially thawed, sprinkle with 1 tablespoon sugar, mash with a fork or potato masher, and set aside until you're topping the shortcakes.

If you're using fresh berries instead of the Ugly Fruit Jam, place the berries in a bowl and sprinkle with 1 tablespoon sugar. Mash with a fork or potato masher and side aside until you're topping the shortcakes.

Healthy Kitchen Hack: Go green with your shortcakes! Since these cornbread-style shortcakes aren't overly sweet, herbed versions also work well as savory sides to serve with chilis, soup, salads, or our Cheesy Broccoli and Greens Soup with Za'atar (page 121), Spicy Red Lentil and Chorizo Stew (page 238) or Oregano, Fennel, and Garlic Slow Cooker Pulled Pork (page 241). Simply mix in a combo of ½ cup chopped fresh basil, parsley, cilantro, dill, chives, thyme, and/or rosemary with the dry ingredients.

Per Serving (using Ugly Fruit Jam and vanilla Greek yogurt): Calories 247; Total Fat: 7g; Saturated Fat: 1g; Cholesterol: 34mg; Sodium: 127mg; Total Carbohydrates: 44g; Fiber: 2g; Protein: 7g

Chocolate Tahini Pudding Cups

SERVES 4

Prep time: 5 minutes, plus 15 minutes for setting

Cook time: 10 minutes

1 cup fresh, frozen, or canned fruit (sliced or chopped if large)

¼ cup tahini, divided

3 tablespoons cornstarch

3 tablespoons sugar

2 tablespoons unsweetened cocoa powder

¼ teaspoon kosher or sea salt

2 cups 2% milk

1 teaspoon vanilla extract

⅛ teaspoon smoked paprika (optional)

You'll never go back to the boxed stuff once you discover how easy it is to make superior-quality chocolate pudding at home. This handy recipe can be whipped up anytime, as it relies on pantry and refrigerator staples, and you can use up whatever fruit you have on hand, like fresh in-season apple slices, canned mandarin oranges, frozen berries, or even dried fruit—get creative! Our Mediterranean flavor twists include the indispensable Middle Eastern staple, tahini, along with a hint of smoky spice, if you desire (which we are now also loving in our desserts like our Smoked Paprika Peanut Butter Oatmeal Cookies on page 266).

Divide the fruit among four 5- or 6-ounce ramekins. Drizzle 1 teaspoon tahini over the fruit in each ramekin. Set aside.

In a medium saucepan over medium heat, whisk together the cornstarch, sugar, cocoa, and salt. Slowly whisk in the milk and continue to whisk until all the dry ingredients are incorporated. Cook, whisking frequently, until the pudding starts to thicken, 4 to 5 minutes. Turn the heat to medium-low and whisk constantly for an additional 1 to 2 minutes until fairly thick. Remove from the heat and whisk in the remaining tahini, vanilla, and smoked paprika if desired. Carefully pour the pudding over the fruit in the four ramekins. Cool for 15 minutes, then serve at room temperature or cover the ramekins and chill in the refrigerator for at least 1 hour before serving.

Healthy Kitchen Hack: For future batches of this pudding (because we know you'll be making it again!), switch it up with some of these fruit and spice combo ideas: pears + grated nutmeg, oranges + ground ginger, cherries + ¼ teaspoon almond extract. Or whisk a few tablespoons of our Ugly Fruit Jam (page 259) into the pudding, once removed from the stove.

Per Serving: Calories: 214; Total Fat: 9g; Saturated Fat: 3g; Cholesterol: 10mg; Sodium: 209mg; Total Carbohydrates: 26g; Fiber: 3g; Protein: 7g

Five-Day Meal Plans

	GLUTEN-FREE	VEGETARIAN	SEAFOOD TWICE A WEEK	MEATLESS MONDAY
MONDAY				
Breakfast	Spiced Turkish Coffee Coffee Cake 39 (make on the weekend with gluten-free oats)	Spiced Turkish Coffee Coffee Cake 39 (make on the weekend)	Spiced Turkish Coffee Coffee Cake 39 (make on the weekend)	Spiced Turkish Coffee Coffee Cake 39 (make on the weekend)
Lunch	Honey, Orange, and Scallion Vinaigrette 70 over Romaine (save half of dressing), hard-boiled eggs (make on the weekend), plain Greek yogurt with fruit and seeds	Honey, Orange, and Scallion Vinaigrette 70 over Romaine (save half of dressing), hard-boiled eggs (make on the weekend), plain Greek yogurt with fruit and seeds	Honey, Orange, and Scallion Vinaigrette 70 over Romaine (save half of dressing), hard-boiled eggs (make on the weekend), plain Greek yogurt with fruit and seeds	Honey, Orange, and Scallion Vinaigrette 70 over Romaine (save half of dressing), hard-boiled eggs (make on the weekend), plain Greek yogurt with fruit and seeds
Snack	Pumpkin Hummus 63 with gluten-free crackers, fruit	Pumpkin Hummus 63 with whole-grain crackers, fruit	Pumpkin Hummus 63 with whole-grain crackers, fruit	Pumpkin Hummus 63 with whole-grain crackers, fruit
Dinner	Sheet Pan Sesame Seed Fish with Baby Potatoes 205, Windowsill Herb Salad with Tomatoes and Za'atar 76	Zucchini, Carrot, and Gorgonzola Patties 173, with raw vegetables (make extra za'atar dressing for dipping), cooked barley	Sheet Pan Sesame Seed Fish with Baby Potatoes 205, Windowsill Herb Salad with Tomatoes and Za'atar 76	Zucchini, Carrot, and Gorgonzola Patties 173, with raw vegetables (make extra za'atar dressing for dipping), cooked barley
Dessert	Chocolate Orange Mug Cake 264 (make with gluten-free flour)	Chocolate Orange Mug Cake 264	Chocolate Orange Mug Cake 264	Chocolate Orange Mug Cake 264
TUESDAY				
Breakfast	Leftover Spiced Turkish Coffee Coffee Cake 39	Leftover Spiced Turkish Coffee Coffee Cake 39	Leftover Spiced Turkish Coffee Coffee Cake 39	Leftover Spiced Turkish Coffee Coffee Cake 39
Lunch	Israeli Couscous "Pasta Salad" 85 (make with GF couscous or other pasta) with leftover Honey, Orange, and Scallion Vinaigrette 70	Israeli Couscous "Pasta Salad" 85 with leftover Honey, Orange, and Scallion Vinaigrette 70	Israeli Couscous "Pasta Salad" 85 with leftover Honey, Orange, and Scallion Vinaigrette 70	Israeli Couscous "Pasta Salad" 85 with leftover Honey, Orange, and Scallion Vinaigrette 70
Snack	Vanilla and Fruit Seeded Granola Bars 66 (make 1–2 days ahead with gluten-free oats)	Vanilla and Fruit Seeded Granola Bars 66 (make 1–2 days ahead)	Vanilla and Fruit Seeded Granola Bars 66 (make 1–2 days ahead)	Vanilla and Fruit Seeded Granola Bars 66 (make 1–2 days ahead)
Dinner	Stuffed Greek Lamb Burgers 233 wrapped in lettuce leaf, raw vegetables served with extra Mediterranean Mayo 235	Cauliflower Steaks with Sun-Dried Tomato and Basil Pesto 175, stove-top polenta with extra pesto	Stuffed Greek Lamb Burgers 233 wrapped in lettuce leaf, raw vegetables served with extra Mediterranean Mayo 235	Stuffed Greek Lamb Burgers 233 wrapped in lettuce leaf, raw vegetables served with extra Mediterranean Mayo 235
Dessert	Lemon Ricotta No-Churn Gelato 268 (make up to a week ahead)	Lemon Ricotta No-Churn Gelato 268 (make up to a week ahead)	Lemon Ricotta No-Churn Gelato 268 (make up to a week ahead)	Lemon Ricotta No-Churn Gelato 268 (make up to a week ahead)
WEDNESDAY				
Breakfast	Lentil, Greens, and Parmesan Frittata 37 (optional to make night before)	Lentil, Greens, and Parmesan Frittata 37 (optional to make night before)	Lentil, Greens, and Parmesan Frittata 37 (optional to make night before)	Lentil, Greens, and Parmesan Frittata 37 (optional to make night before)

	GLUTEN-FREE	VEGETARIAN	SEAFOOD TWICE A WEEK	MEATLESS MONDAY
Lunch	Very Veggie Sustainable Soup for One 111, gluten-free crackers, Roasted Cabbage Wedge Caesar Salad with gluten-free croutons 78	Very Veggie Sustainable Soup for One 111, crackers, Roasted Cabbage Wedge Caesar Salad 78 (Hack variation made with Gorgonzola Cheese Dressing)	Very Veggie Sustainable Soup for One 111, crackers, Roasted Cabbage Wedge Caesar Salad 78	Very Veggie Sustainable Soup for One 111, crackers, Roasted Cabbage Wedge Caesar Salad 78
Snack	Baklava-Flavored Frozen Yogurt Bark 262 (make day before)	Baklava-Flavored Frozen Yogurt Bark 262 (make day before)	Baklava-Flavored Frozen Yogurt Bark 262 (make day before)	Baklava-Flavored Frozen Yogurt Bark 262 (make day before)
Dinner	Lemon Chicken Tenders with Capers 244 (make with gluten-free flour), carrot sticks	"Not Quite Paella" Farro Medley 186, Windowsill Herb Salad with Tomatoes and Za'atar 76	Lemon Chicken Tenders with Capers 244, crusty bread, carrot sticks	Lemon Chicken Tenders with Capers 244, crusty bread, carrot sticks
Dessert	Minty Melon Mimosa Cups 261 or plain fruit	Minty Melon Mimosa Cups 261 or plain fruit	Minty Melon Mimosa Cups 261 or plain fruit	Minty Melon Mimosa Cups 261 or plain fruit

THURSDAY

	GLUTEN-FREE	VEGETARIAN	SEAFOOD TWICE A WEEK	MEATLESS MONDAY
Breakfast	Leftover Lentil, Greens, and Parmesan Frittata 37	Leftover Lentil, Greens, and Parmesan Frittata 37	Leftover Lentil, Greens, and Parmesan Frittata 37	Leftover Lentil, Greens, and Parmesan Frittata 37
Lunch	Leftover Chicken Tenders with Capers 244, leftover Roasted Cabbage Wedge Caesar Salad 78, fruit	Leftover "Not Quite Paella" Farro Medley 186, leftover Roasted Cabbage Wedge Caesar Salad 78, fruit	Leftover Chicken Tenders with Capers 244, leftover Roasted Cabbage Wedge Caesar Salad 78, fruit	Leftover Chicken Tenders with Capers 244, leftover Roasted Cabbage Wedge Caesar Salad 78, fruit
Snack	Antipasto Pickles 52 (make day before) with a locally produced cheese	Antipasto Pickles 52 (make day before) with a locally produced cheese	Antipasto Pickles 52 (make day before) with a locally produced cheese	Antipasto Pickles 52 (make day before) with a locally produced cheese
Dinner	Microwaved White Fish with Tomatoes and Chives 198, Tahini Use-Up-Those-Veggies Slaw 75 (optional to make day before)	Roasted Thyme Mushrooms over Parmesan Polenta Squares 193, Tahini Use-Up-Those-Veggies Slaw 75 (optional to make day before)	Microwaved White Fish with Tomatoes and Chives 198, Tahini Use-Up-Those-Veggies Slaw 75 (optional to make day before)	Microwaved White Fish with Tomatoes and Chives 198, Tahini Use-Up-Those-Veggies Slaw 75 (optional to make day before)
Dessert	A few pieces of dark chocolate	A few pieces of dark chocolate	A few pieces of dark chocolate	A few pieces of dark chocolate

FRIDAY

	GLUTEN-FREE	VEGETARIAN	SEAFOOD TWICE A WEEK	MEATLESS MONDAY
Breakfast	Good Morning Polenta with Ricotta and Apples 30	Good Morning Polenta with Ricotta and Apples 30	Good Morning Polenta with Ricotta and Apples 30	Good Morning Polenta with Ricotta and Apples 30
Lunch	Red Pepper Breakfast Biscuits (made with GF flour) with eggs to make sandwiches 33 (make night before), paired with salad greens	Red Pepper Breakfast Biscuits with eggs to make sandwiches 33 (make night before), paired with salad greens	Red Pepper Breakfast Biscuits with eggs to make sandwiches 33 (make night before), paired with salad greens	Red Pepper Breakfast Biscuits with eggs to make sandwiches 33 (make night before), paired with salad greens
Snack	Lemon, Black Pepper, and Honey Toasted Walnuts 51 (make extra for Cheese Board)	Lemon, Black Pepper, and Honey Toasted Walnuts 51 (make extra for Cheese Board)	Lemon, Black Pepper, and Honey Toasted Walnuts 51 (make extra for Cheese Board)	Lemon, Black Pepper, and Honey Toasted Walnuts 51 (make extra for Cheese Board)
Dinner	Toasted Squash Seeds and Cheese Board 61 paired with smoked fishes, gluten-free crackers, as dinner-sized	Toasted Squash Seeds and Cheese Board 61 paired with Lemon Hummus 231, as dinner-sized	Toasted Squash Seeds and Cheese Board 61 paired with Lemon Hummus 231, as dinner-sized	Toasted Squash Seeds and Cheese Board 61 paired with Lemon Hummus 231, as dinner-sized
Dessert	Chocolate Tahini Pudding Cups 273	Chocolate Tahini Pudding Cups 273	Chocolate Tahini Pudding Cups 273	Chocolate Tahini Pudding Cups 273

Acknowledgments

To Clare Pelino and Claire Schulz, who brought our vision for this book to life. To Elise Cellucci, who turned her home kitchen into a magical food photography studio for our recipes. To our rockstar marketing team, headed up by Lindsay Marshall, the amazing eyes and vision of art director Sarah Avinger, and the diligence and creativity of production editor Jessika Rieck for graciously accepting our many, many edits and requests.. And most importantly to our dear families, trusted friends, loyal followers, and very vocal recipe testers—this cookbook is dedicated to all of you. XO

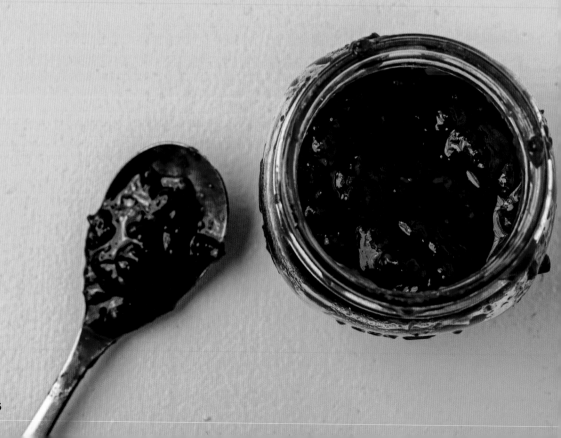

Index

About
the Authors

Serena Ball, MS, RD, and Deanna Segrave-Daly, RD, each have more than twenty years of culinary nutrition experience and have dedicated their careers to helping people make delicious and nutritious meals. Together, they are the authors of *The 30-Minute Mediterranean Diet Cookbook* and the *Easy Everyday Mediterranean Diet Cookbook*. Deanna lives in Philadelphia with her husband and daughter, and Serena lives outside St. Louis with her husband and five children. You can find them online at teaspoonofspice.com and doing weekly live-stream recipe demonstrations on their Facebook page, Teaspoon of Spice.